Ophthalmic N

ITS PRACTICE AND

F. C. E. Rooke SRN OND
Senior Nursing Officer,
St Paul's Eye Hospital, Liverpool

P. J. Rothwell SRN OND
Ophthalmic Nurse Tutor,
St Paul's Eye Hospital, Liverpool

D. F. Woodhouse FRCS
Consultant Ophthalmologist,
Wolverhampton and Midland Counties Eye Infirmary, Wolverhampton

CHURCHILL LIVINGSTONE
EDINBURGH LONDON AND NEW YORK 1980

CHURCHILL LIVINGSTONE
Medical Division of the Longman Group Limited

Distributed in the United States of America by Churchill
Livingstone Inc., 19 West 44th Street, New York,
N.Y. 10036, and by associated companies, branches and
representatives throughout the world.

First published 1980

ISBN 0 443 01494 9

British Library Cataloguing in Publication Data
Rooke, F C E
  Ophthalmic nursing.
  1. Ophthalmic nursing
  I. Title   II. Rothwell, P J
  III. Woodhouse, D F
  610.73'677   RE88   79-40865

Printed in Singapore by Kua Co., Book Manufacturer, Pte Ltd

Preface

This textbook aims to be a comprehensive account of the practice of ophthalmic nursing and its need has arisen from the development of this speciality of nursing since the inception of the Ophthalmic Nursing Board in 1952. Through a system of examinations and recognised ophthalmic nurse training schools, the board has helped to produce a nationally accepted standard of nursing practice in the British Isles. There are now over five thousand nurses registered with the board, and recently an advanced diploma course for the more senior ophthalmic nurse has been approved.

Several smaller textbooks on ophthalmic nursing have long been available; some of these give sufficient detail on the nursing aspects, while introducing ophthalmological knowledge, which is usually better studied in some of the standard textbooks (see Bibliography). It is recommended that the student use one of these in conjunction with the present work, especially in preparing for examinations.

The work is written to include the needs of both nurses first beginning ophthalmic work and also for more experienced nurses. Although it will include elementary principles well known to the latter, it is hoped that the format will be of interest to them when teaching. It includes sufficient detail of nursing techniques to give a foundation to those beginning their studies of ophthalmic nursing and it also covers a wide area of application from the hospital departments to the community. Teaching is a responsibility of all experienced nurses; in a rapidly evolving technology such as nursing, it is important that teaching is based as much in the clinical area as in the school.

This book should both inform and stimulate interest in the fascinating aspect of ophthalmic nursing. Man is a seeing animal and has used vision to create civilisation as we know it, as well as to communicate with his fellows. Nursing is concerned with the caring support of patients in illness and disease, and as the eye is but part of the patient, so the ophthalmic nurse must be a complete nurse with special skills and understanding. The authors have received inspiration particularly from Mrs M. B. Carmichael and the late Miss M. P. Jones, who each served on the Ophthalmic Nursing Board as secretaries between 1952 and 1975.

In writing this book the authors have been conscious of a readership wider than that of the student ophthalmic nurse and have included material which should be of interest to the more senior and responsible members of the nursing profession. The book may be of interest to:

1. The student ophthalmic nurse who may wish to base a specialised training on the fundamentals of nursing theory and practice, but will not be immediately concerned with the administrative and educational matters.

2. The senior ophthalmic nurse who wishes to apply the practice of nursing within the organisation of hospital and clinic and requires both a management skill and a knowledge of the planning and acquiring of essential facilities.

3. Other nurses such as tutors and administrators who wish to learn something of the way in which ophthalmic nursing is organised within the context of the United Kingdom as well as its practical methods.

It is obvious that certain sections, especially those on education and management, have been kept to a minimum and give an ophthalmic emphasis to supplement the details available in those books quoted in the Bibliography.

The authors are also indebted to our illustrator, Mrs Price, and to Miss Emmerson, who, on behalf of the Publishers, has done so much to make our work presentable. We are also most grateful to Mrs Ascott, who has typed and retyped our manuscript. We have received encouragement and guidance from those colleagues who have read parts of the manuscript but realise that this type of book will have omissions, for which we alone are responsible; we hope that interested readers will let us know of these.

The authors acknowledge permission to use illustrations of equipment from the various companies named and of stationery from the Wolverhampton Area Health Authority (WAHA).

Wolverhampton, 1980   F. C. E. R
                                                     P. J. R
                                                     D. F. W

Contents

Nursing procedures – care of patient
                  – anaesthetic
                  – post-operative
Ophthalmic surgical instruments
Electrical equipment and its care
Use of magnet

1

Introduction

NURSING AND OPHTHALMOLOGY

Nursing is a satisfying profession in which the knowledge of the nurse is applied for the needs of patients. In ophthalmic nursing specialised knowledge is required for the needs of the eye and vision, but the nurse still requires to exercise her basic skills of general nursing as the eye is only part of the patient, who, especially if elderly, may have a number of general diseases. As many of us value sight almost as much as life itself, there is much satisfaction in ministering to those whose vision is threatened by disease. The nurse must at all time exercise her skill with sympathy and an understanding of the problems faced by someone whose eyesight is threatened or becoming progressively worse.

Ophthalmic nursing also demands accuracy of judgment and of manual dexterity as the eye is both small and easily damaged. All nursing procedures on the eye need to be performed with precision and a light touch, always avoiding any pressure on the eye through the eyelids. Ophthalmic instruments are necessarily fine and easily damaged and the nurse will develop the special skills required for the cleaning and care of such instruments.

In spite of requiring specialised skills and knowledge, the ophthalmic nurse finds that the field of ophthalmic nursing is by no means narrow. On the surgical side it extends from the new born with congenital defects or squint, to the aged patients with cataract or glaucoma. Between these there are conditions such as injury and retinal detachment which may require surgery and can occur at any age. Most eye patients never require surgery and the need for the care of medical conditions of the eye extends from those conditions, such as conjunctivitis, which require purely local treatment, to those eye conditions which arise as part of a generalised disease such as diabetes or hypertension. Even conjunctivitis may arise as a result of a generalised infection with, for instance, staphylococcus or herpes simplex. Ophthalmology is a speciality with many links to general medicine and the nurse will find many of the basic skills required in the general course of training as important as in any other field of nursing. Ophthalmic nursing presents many challenges to the skill of the nurse, who should find enjoyment and satisfaction in the practice of her profession. The development of courses leading to specialised qualifications has helped her to minister to the needs of these patients at a standard required by contemporary knowledge. The progressive development of further knowledge will present greater demands but also the greater satisfaction of being able to accomplish more for the patient.

Principles of this book

Any textbook must teach by its content, much of this being the facts of the subject. But a book on nursing, a practical technology, should also teach method; the methods of learning from experience in nursing by observation, by the proper recording of observed data, and by the forward planning of nursing techniques and the testing of these techniques. 'Life is short, the Art long' (Hippocrates), and these methods can be time-wasting or time-saving; this book will show the importance of efficient methods for the recording of nursing data in learning and in clinical practice.

Writing is not the only medium for records, and just as numbers are used in measurement, simple anatomical diagrams (like those used in this book) can also be the best way of recording spatial relations and the position of structures.

The basic sciences of nursing, as with medicine, are usually regarded as anatomy, physiology and pathology. Anatomy and physiology are described in Chapter 2 in a unified form since structure and function have evolved together. Dull as anatomy tends to be when considered in its details, it does introduce much of the vocabulary which will be used in the descriptions of ophthalmic disease and nursing in the other chapters. The student beginning ophthalmic nursing is urged to study this chapter together with illustrated books and atlases (see Bibliography) and models, not forgetting a human skull and the living subject. The more experienced nurse can use this chapter to revise the anatomical and physiological foundations of ophthalmic nursing and should be able to relate them to clinical experience.

The chapters on ophthalmic nursing practice and techniques, the care and sterilisation of instruments, ophthalmic drugs, and ophthalmic nursing management all have a wide application and should be referred to as necessary. The remaining chapters introduce the subject matter in relation to those departments of an eye clinic where the experience is most likely to be needed; there will inevitably be some overlap and the student looking for some detail of ophthalmic nursing should use either the glossary or index.

It is hoped that an experienced nurse will be able to read the text as a whole, with interest and some enjoyment. The student beginning ophthalmic nursing is warned not to read too far ahead of her experience. Learning can be accomplished by discovery as much as by imitation and habit; too much reading can make the mind insensitive to discoveries, through which the knowledge required for nursing may be extended. This book will refer to many established and accepted nursing procedures; as much as they are commended to the student, they have themselves evolved through years of practice and the conscious reduction of error, so that it is certain that they will continue to be improved. Innovation is essential in the progress of nursing, but it has to pass strict tests of clinical advantage, acceptability and, not least, economics.

Principles of ophthalmic nursing

Ophthalmic nursing shares the basic principles of all nursing based on the clinical care of patients within a professional relationship, both to the patient himself and to other professions involved, especially the doctor. Florence Nightingale, in her *Notes on Nursing*, described nursing as the assistance of 'the reparative process which Nature has instituted and which we call disease'. In 1859 this would have been a new idea; death and disease had been traditionally set against life and health. It was only in the previous year that the German physician Virchow had, in his *Cellular Pathology*, finally overthrown Galenic medicine and established the cell as both the unit of biological life and of disease. The cell is the unit at which life exists and by which, as the *gamete*, it is passed to succeeding generations. Death occurs essentially at a cellular level and death also ends the progress of disease.

Disease as a concept was defined by Virchow when he discussed it at the level of the cell and the observed microscopic changes which occur in the cell during various clinical diseases. The cell contains the biochemistry required to create the energy used by the body in growth and survival, and it should be understood that some cells (especially epithelial) maintain a potential for multiplication throughout the life of the body, although others (such as the nerve cells in the central nervous system, including the retina) do not. Cellular multiplication in some diseases (such as cancer) is progressively harmfull, but in most diseases it helps to repair the tissues either by replacing the cells by their own type or by fibrous (scar) tissue. Florence Nightingale's concept of disease as reparative may not be universally true, but it is true enough to form a basis for many nursing objectives. It is a foundation for the nursing care of surgical patients, as the physiological processes are active in the recovery of the patient from surgical trauma, which may be general (such as surgical shock due to blood loss) or local (such as the healing of the surgical wound). The nursing care is aimed to support the physiology of recovery and to protect the injured or diseased part of the body.

Ophthalmic nursing as the nursing of patients with eye diseases and symptoms, requires an understanding of the structure and function of the eye and related organs as well as the relationship to the body as a whole. Much of this knowledge is required for the intelligent planning of the nursing care of the patient. Clinical experience will allow this knowledge at a biological level to be integrated with the psychological and sociological aspects of the patients' problems. It is convenient to structure knowledge into categories such as the chemical, biological, psychological or sociological aspect of disease, but practical nursing in the clinic requires a balanced ability to use all these facets of knowledge; success in nursing depends on the nurse's ability to use all her knowledge and experience as a whole and an over-specialised knowledge does not necessarily produce the best nursing.

An example may emphasise the interaction of these elements in disease. A patient aged 27 years has rapidly deteriorating vision due to bilateral cataract. The immediate cause of his symptoms is clearly due to the cataract, which is an opacity of the lens of each eye, so that his anxiety may be relieved by explaining the curative nature of his condition. It is then proved that the cataract is due to diabetes mellitus, a disorder of carbohydrate metabolism and deficiency of insulin; his anxiety will be increased and he will require reassurance that, although diabetes is a chronic disease, he will be able to control it with diet and treatment and return to useful employment. However, he will not be able to measure his injections of insulin for himself, let alone work, until he can see, so that cataract surgery becomes more urgent; the need for this and the good chances of success also require explanation. The diabetes requires control, the cataracts surgery, and the patient will then require spectacles and possibly rehabilitation for a new job. All this requires time and the medical staff will explain this both to the patient and nursing staff. The nurse, being at the centre of the continuous care of the patient, will need to plan the nursing well ahead, provide psychological support for the patient's temporary insecurity, and identify the need for further specialised help and support survices, such as occupational therapy and medical social welfare. Techniques used in nurse care planning will be detailed in Chapter 3.

History of ophthalmic nursing

The history of disease and medical practice is as old as recorded history and many of the words used in ophthalmology, e.g. *chalazion*, *cataract* and *glaucoma*, come from the medicine of Classical Greece.

The Royal London Ophthalmic Hospital, later Moorfields, was established after the Napoleonic war, when there were many of the London poor, often disbanded soldiers and sailors, with injuries and diseases of the eye. Following the Egyptian campaign, *trachoma* became endemic. In 1846 Sir William Bowman joined the staff of this hospital and devoted his attention wholly to diseases of the eyes and was one of the first to use the new ophthalmoscope, developed by Helmholtz in 1851. As well as being the founder of British ophthalmology, Sir William Bowman understood the need for nurses to be professionally trained. In 1847 he established St. John's House, from which the pupil-nurses attended King's College Hospital for instruction by the medical staff, and in 1856 the Order took over the nursing at the hospital 'so as to introduce a higher class of nurse and a better system of nursing into the wards of the hospital'. The professional basis of nursing was endorsed by the establishment of similar schools of nursing, especially the Nightingale School at the new St Thomas's Hospital in 1860.

As the standards of nursing care improved, it became obvious that a national standard of training controlled by a statutory body was required and in 1919 a Nurse Registration Act set up nationally recognised examinations and a State Register, although a three-year course of training had been recommended from 1892. In spite of the fact that an ophthalmologist originally identified the need for professionally trained nurses, no national standard for ophthalmic nursing was established until 1952, when a group of ophthalmic nurses and ophthalmic consultants met together and formed the Ophthalmic Nursing Board. This Board is a non-statutory body but it has set up standards of ophthalmic nursing practice and education which have been accepted throughout the British Isles. Its qualification is accepted for membership of the International Ophthalmic Association, which is independent of the Board and represents the views of its members.

2

The normal eye

Anatomy of the eye
Eye as self-contained system
Eye as dependent on the human body
Eye as part of a visual system
Psychological aspects of vision

The study of anatomy and physiology is essential to the understanding of the normal healthy eye so that the changes which occur with disease may also be understood. This chapter is an introduction to the structure of the eye and its related tissues and to its function as man's most important sensory organ. The parts described should be identified as far as possible in the living body; other parts not visible without dissection can be identified on a human skull, X-ray film and class-room anatomical models. The ophthalmoscope is a specialised diagnostic instrument, but the student nurse can learn to use it sufficiently well to appreciate the view it gives of the eye through the pupil and how its invention in 1851 led to the development of ophthalmology as a speciality.

The eye develops its structure around the retina for the needs of vision. The retina is part of the central nervous system and is one of the earliest parts to become structurally different in the early development of the embryo. As an optic cup, the retinal element buds out from the central nervous system, and this bud eventually forms the retina, optic nerve and the posterior layers of the iris and ciliary body. As with the rest of the central nervous system, the retina is composed mainly of neurones (nerve cells) and of neuroglia (connective tissue) and its nerve fibres do not regenerate if damaged. The optic cup exercises a chemical control on the development of the other tissues of the eye as has been shown in experimental animals by transplanting it to other parts of the embryo where eye structures will then develop.

THE VISIBLE EYE

The eye is a spherical organ 2·5 cm in diameter, but only those parts of it exposed by the palpebral fissure, between the margins of the upper and lower eyelids, are usually visible, More of the eye can be exposed during examination by drawing away the eyelids and asking the patient to vary his gaze (see Figure 2.1).

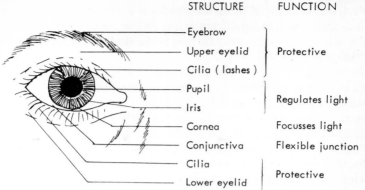

STRUCTURE	FUNCTION
Eyebrow	
Upper eyelid	Protective
Cilia (lashes)	
Pupil	
Iris	Regulates light
Cornea	Focusses light
Conjunctiva	Flexible junction
Cilia	
Lower eyelid	Protective

Fig. 2.1 Visible eye

The lids are dermal folds, specially modified for the protection of the eye. On their outer surfaces they present a covering of delicate and loosely attached skin; on their inner side they present a delicate mucous membrane, the conjunctiva, which is reflected from the lids on to the exposed front of the eyeball. Everywhere the membrane is transparent, so that the underlying vessels and glands and the colour of the sclera can be clearly seen. The conjunctiva forms the deep fold (fornix) between the eyelids and the eye, which can therefore move freely and independently of the eyelid movements; the conjunctiva is moistened by the tear fluid from the lacrimal gland as well as by mucous glands. The eyelids are protective and the regular blinking maintains a moist film over the exposed surface of the eye (cornea and conjunctiva). Note that the skin of the eyelids is thin and (except for the lashes and eyebrows) almost hairless, this gives it mobility although it can also stretch and become swollen to a great size as over an ecchymosis (black eye). The disc formed by the iris and perforated by the pupil regulates the entry of light into the eye, needed for vision. The iris is attached peripherally to the middle of the anterior surface of the ciliary body, which is not visible, and projects forward a little towards its centre where it rests upon the lens, separating the anterior from the posterior chamber; it also contains the muscles which by their contraction and relaxation regulate the size of the pupil (see Figure 2.14). The limbus is the border between the sclera (white of eye) with overlying conjunctiva and the clear cornea (window of eye, anterior to pupil and iris).

THE ORBIT

Study bones by (1) macerated skull, (2) palpation of bones on living subject, and (3) x-ray of skull. The reader is warned that some plastic replica-skulls contain significant errors in the bones of the orbit.

The orbit is the bony cavity formed in the skull around the eye and has two functions:

1. Protection for the eye and its adnexa.
2. Communication between face and cranium for:
   Nerve of face (ophthalmic from Gasserian ganglion).
   Veins of face and cranium joining via orbital veins.
   Arteries anastomose via ophthalmic artery to carotid.

Form: orbit is pyramidal or pear-shaped (see Fig. 2.2); it has four walls, of which the medial walls are parallel and the lateral walls are at an angle of 90 degrees to each other.

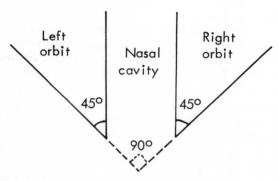

Fig. 2.2 Relationship between orbits

Walls of bone, thicker in front where orbit joins face (orbital margin) and thinner behind.

Bones: hard connective tissue consisting of:

1. Calcium salts – contributing to hardness.
2. Protein in the form of collagen fibres – binding the calcium salts, and
3. Bone cells – the living part of bone.

Seven bones help to form each orbit, four of which are filled by nasal air sinuses (see Fig. 2.3).

The air sinuses:

1. lighten the bones;
2. make voice more resonant;
3. may become infected (sinusitis).

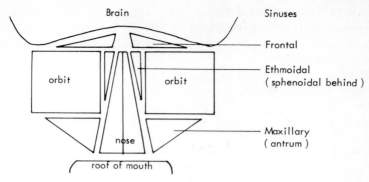

Fig. 2.3 Orbit, nose and sinuses

Boundaries of orbit – roof, floor and two walls (see Fig. 2.4).
1. Roof (see Fig. 2.5).
  Note: fossa for lacrimal gland, bone thin and translucent.

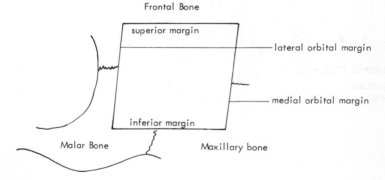

Fig. 2.4 Orbital boundaries

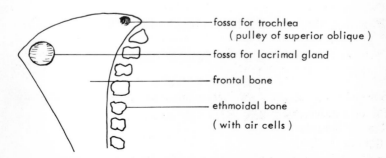

Fig. 2.5 Roof of orbit

2. Lateral Wall (see Fig. 2.6).
Note: superior orbital fissure for nerves and vessels.

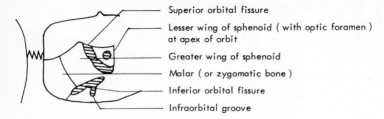

Superior orbital fissure

Lesser wing of sphenoid (with optic foramen) at apex of orbit

Greater wing of sphenoid

Malar (or zygomatic bone)

Inferior orbital fissure

Infraorbital groove

Fig. 2.6 Lateral wall of orbit

3. Floor (see Fig. 2.7).
Note: infra-orbital fissure (a) and nasolacrimal canal (b).

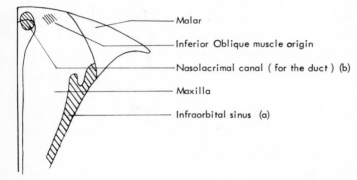

Malar

Inferior Oblique muscle origin

Nasolacrimal canal (for the duct) (b)

Maxilla

Infraorbital sinus (a)

Fig. 2.7 Floor of orbit

4. Medial Wall (see Fig. 2.8).
Note: lacrimal fossa for lacrimal sac, optic foramen for optic nerve and ophthalmic artery.

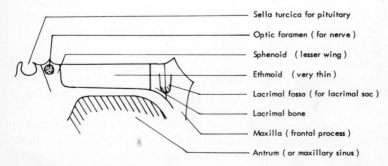

Sella turcica for pituitary

Optic foramen (for nerve)

Sphenoid   (lesser wing)

Ethmoid   (very thin)

Lacrimal fossa (for lacrimal sac)

Lacrimal bone

Maxilla (frontal process)

Antrum (or maxillary sinus)

Fig. 2.8 Medial wall of orbit

Relations of orbit (Fig. 2.3).

1. Above – frontal sinus, cranial fossa, frontal lobe of brain.
2. Below – maxillary sinus (antrum).
3. Nasal – ethmoid sinus, nasal cavity.
4. Temporal – temporal fossa and middle cranial fossa.
5. Behind – sphenoid sinus and middle cranial fossa.

Neurovascular foramina and fissures (Fig. 2.6).
1. Optic foramen.
2. Superior orbital fissure.
3. Inferior orbital fissure.
4. Infra-orbital canal and groove.

Contents of orbit (see Fig. 2.9)

1. Eyeball (globe), optic nerve, ocular muscles and tendons.
2. Tenon's capsule – connective tissue 'socket' for eye-movement.
3. Orbital fat – both inside and outside muscle-cone.
4. Nerves, arteries and veins.
5. Lacrimal gland and lacrimal sac.
6. Periorbita.

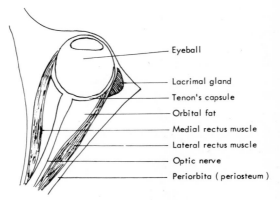

Eyeball

Lacrimal gland

Tenon's capsule

Orbital fat

Medial rectus muscle

Lateral rectus muscle

Optic nerve

Periorbita (periosteum)

Fig. 2.9 Contents of orbit

Most diseases of the orbit produce swelling behind the eye; as the orbit is rigid, protrusion of the eye (proptosis) results. *Proptosis* or *exophthalmos* is a cardinal sign of orbital disease.

The orbit is closed anteriorly by the eyelids and orbital septum. Those arteries and veins connecting the circulation of the face to that of the orbit pass through the orbital septum, which is thin and separates the orbital fat from the tissues of the eyelids.

Orbital vessels

Orbital arteries are branches of the internal carotid via the ophthalmic artery with anastomotic connections to the external carotid through the orbital septum. The branches supply:

1. Eye by posterior and anterior ciliary arteries.
2. Retina by central retinal artery.
3. Muscles by muscular branches.
4. Lacrimal gland by a lacrimal branch.

Orbital veins drain the blood from the orbital structures to the cavernous and pterygoid plexuses and also have anastomotic connection to the face; infection of the face can spread through the orbit to the veins inside the skull.

Ocular muscles

Seven muscles, with six to eye. Four rectus muscles, two oblique, and the levator muscle of the upper eyelid.

Cranial nerves

When learning, describe nerves as follows:

1. Origin, course, and termination of nerve.
2. Position of nerve and its relation to neighbouring structures.
3. Distribution of nerve (muscles, skin, glands, vessels).

Pattern of nervous system (see Fig. 2.10).
This structure of peripheral to central to peripheral nervous activity is the basis for the reflex arc; e.g. knee jerk, corneal reflex, etc.

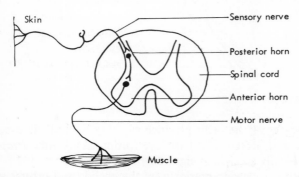

Fig. 2.10 Connection of nervous system (as shown for section of spinal cord)

Central nervous system: Brain, spinal cord, and retina.

Cranial nerves

1. Olfactory (smell).
2. Optic (vision).
3. Oculomotor (eye and upper lid movements).
4. Trochlear (eye movement – superior oblique muscle only).
5. Trigeminal (face sensation and jaw movements).
6. Abducens (eye movement – lateral rectus muscle only).
7. Facial (face movements).
8. Auditory (hearing and position-sensation).
9. Glossopharyngeal   (movement and sensation of
10. Vagus   upper gut and lungs).
11. Accessory (neck and shoulder movement).
12. Hypoglossal (tongue movement).

Orbital nerves

A. *Motor nerves* (3rd, 4th and 6th) all enter by the superior orbital fissure and supply all seven extra-ocular muscles:

3rd nerve (*Oculomotor*) – all extra-ocular muscles except two (those supplied by 4th and 6th); also intraocular sphincter of pupil and ciliary muscle (accommodation).

4th nerve (*trochlear*) – superior oblique muscle; the tendon of the muscle passes through the pulley (trochlea).

6th nerve (*abducens*) – lateral rectus muscle; this abducts the eyeball laterally.

Origin of these nerves – midbrain nuclei in floor of 4th ventricle.

Course of nerves – by cavernous sinus (a major venous confluence behind the orbit) and superior orbital fissure to orbit (see Fig. 2.11).

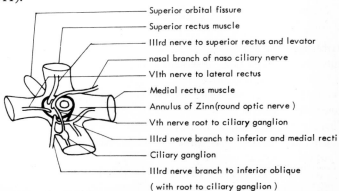

Superior orbital fissure
Superior rectus muscle
IIIrd nerve to superior rectus and levator
nasal branch of naso ciliary nerve
VIth nerve to lateral rectus
Medial rectus muscle
Annulus of Zinn(round optic nerve)
Vth nerve root to ciliary ganglion
IIIrd nerve branch to inferior and medial recti
Ciliary ganglion
IIIrd nerve branch to inferior oblique
(with root to ciliary ganglion)

Fig. 2.11 Orbital distribution of nerves

Termination of nerves – in muscles supplied:
also (3rd nerve) to ciliary ganglion, which supplies ciliary muscle and sphincter muscle of the iris.

B. *Sensory nerves* (2 and 5)
2nd nerve (*optic*) is nerve of eyesight. Fibres from the nasal retina cross over in the chiasma behind the optic foramina (see Fig. 2.12).

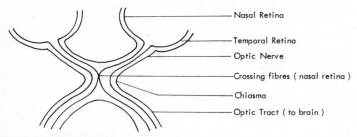

Fig. 2.12 Chiasmal distribution of visual nerve fibres

Origin – nerve fibres arise from retinal ganglion cells.
Termination – nerve ends at chiasma, but nerve fibres continue to pass to lateral geniculate body of brain.
Distribution – visual sensation distributed from lateral geniculate body to occipital cortex.
Other fibres pass to midbrain to form pupil reflexes.
Sheath of optic nerve – this is continuous with membranes of brain (dura, arachnoid, and pia mater); a rise in pressure (hydrocephalus) can cause pressure on nerve and swelling of optic disc (*papilloedema*).
5th nerve (*trigeminal*) – so-called because it has three branches:

1. Ophthalmic.
2. Maxillary.
3. Mandibular.

Distribution (see Fig. 2.13).
Mainly sensation of face, forehead and chin.
Also motor for movement of jaw.
Nerve-cells for sensation lie in the Gasserion ganglion lateral to cavernous sinus.
Three branches radiate from ganglion:
a. *Ophthalmic* itself has three branches, which pass into orbit by superior orbital fissure.
  (i) Lacrimal nerve – mainly to lacrimal gland.
  (ii) Frontal nerve – sensation of upper lid and forehead.
  (iii) Naso-ciliary nerve – sensation of eyeball and front of nose.

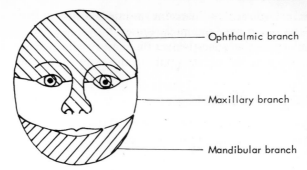

Ophthalmic branch

Maxillary branch

Mandibular branch

Fig. 2.13 Distribution of trigeminal nerve

All three branches supply the upper lid and conjunctiva.
b. *Maxillary* – through foramen rotundum; branches include:

(i) Infraorbital nerve, through the infraorbital fissure to infraorbital foramen. Supplies skin of face from lower eyelid above to upper lip below.
(ii) Zygomatic nerve – supplies skin over lateral side of orbital margin.

c. *Mandibular* – supplies sensation over lower jaw.

C. *Visceral Nerves*
a. *Sympathetic* fibres from superior cervical ganglion via carotid plexus supply:

(i) Dilator of muscle of pupil.
* (ii) Smooth muscle part of levator of upper eyelid.

Paralysis of this nerve causes Horner's syndrome (small pupil, *ptosis* and slight *enophthalmos*).
b. *Parasympathetic* fibres from nucleus of 3rd cranial nerve end in ciliary ganglion, from which new fibres supply the sphincter muscle of the pupil and also the ciliary muscle (the muscle of accommodation).

D. *Facial nerve* – leaves brain with auditory nerve and reaches the lower jaw just below lobule of external ear (pinna). Here it divides into many branches to supply muscles of face, including:

1. Orbicularis oculi muscle – the eye squeezer.
2. Frontalis muscle – the eyebrow raiser.

Anaesthetic facial nerve block is used before intraocular operations to prevent squeezing of the eyelids. A local anaesthetic such as lignocaine or bupivacaine (marcaine) is injected just in front of the tragus of the ear or over the molar bone.

Retrobular injection anaesthetizes the sensory nerves to the eyeball as well as blocking the nerve supply to the extraocular muscles.

THE EYEBALL (Fig. 2.14)

Visible parts – sclera, which is seen through the transparent conjunctiva, cornea, iris, pupil (see page 7).

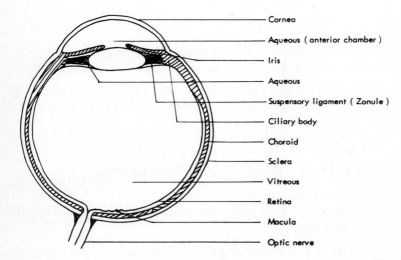

Cornea
Aqueous (anterior chamber)
Iris
Aqueous
Suspensory ligament (Zonule)
Ciliary body
Choroid
Sclera
Vitreous
Retina
Macula
Optic nerve

Fig. 2.14 Structure of the eye

Principles
1. Retina is an offshoot of the brain.
2. Camera construction is based upon the eyeball.
3. Eyeball is a living organ.

Main structure – eyeball has three layers:
1. Outer protective coat – sclera and cornea.
2. Middle vascular layer – choroid, ciliary body and iris.
3. Inner light-sensitive layer – retina.
Inside these layers are three transparent media:
1. Lens – attached to ciliary body by zonule.
2. Aqueous – fluid of anterior segment.
3. Vitreous – gel of posterior segment.
The fourth transparent medium is the cornea.

Sclera – white, and composed of dense fibrous connective tissue, forming the 'skeleton' of the eye. It varies in thickness, with a thick ring anterior to the rectus muscle insertions (Fig. 2.15). It is thinnest deep to rectus muscles.

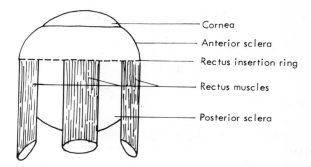

Fig. 2.15 Rectus muscle insertions

The scleral apertures and their contents:

1. Posterior – optic nerve and ciliary arteries and nerves.
2. Equator – venae vorticosae; one from each quadrant.
3. Anterior – anterior ciliary vessels to ciliary body; aqueous veins from the Canal of Schlemm.

The Canal of Schlemm is a narrow canal in the corneo–scleral junction and it forms a ring, draining the aqueous fluid from the eye. Short collecting vessels in the limbus convey the aqueous into the intrascleral plexus whence it drains to the episcleral plexus and the orbital veins; in this efferent plexus there are veins containing blood and others aqueous, until mixture occurs in the larger veins.

The sclera resists internal and external pressure. In glaucoma the intraocular pressure is increased and the sclera gives at the optic nerve, where it is weakest, to produce cupping of the optic disc. In children the sclera is more elastic and *glaucoma* enlarges the eye (*buphthalmos*).

Cornea – this is the anterior sixth of the fibrous layer and is about 12 mm in diameter; it is 0·5 mm thick at the centre and 1 mm at the periphery. It is a convex structure and thus acts as a lens to refract rays of light, producing about 60 per cent of the focusing power of the eye. Corneal structure (five layers) (see Fig. 2.16).

1. *Epithelium* forms the anterior layer, continuous with conjunctiva. Consists of five layers of epithelial cells, becoming flatter as they near the surface.

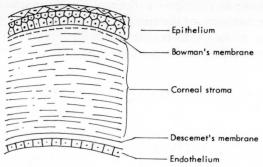

Fig. 2.16 Corneal structure

2. *Bowman's membrane* is the smooth surface of substantia propria, but if destroyed it never regenerates to a smooth surface. Damage to the epithelium alone can heal without scar or opacity.
3. *Substantia propria* is connective tissue and forms nine-tenths of corneal thickness. Collagen-fibres are parallel to surface and the even structure helps to maintain the corneal transparency. It is continuous with the sclera at the limbus.
4. *Descemet's membrane* is a clear elastic layer, resistant to infection. If ulcer present, its base may stretch and bulge to form a descemetocoele.
5. *Endothelium* is a single layer of epithelial cells, which extend over the trabelulae of the angle of the anterior chamber (see Fig. 2.17).

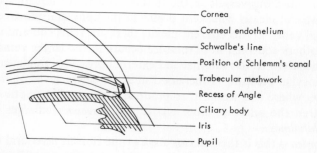

Fig. 2.17 Angle of anterior chamber

Blood supply is normally restricted to peripheral one millimetre; further vascularisation (corneal pannus) may result from disease (*corneal ulcer, trachoma, interstial keratitis,* etc.). Nerve supply for sensation is trigeminal (ophthalmic branch) and the cornea is very sensitive.

Optic properties of cornea depend on its transparency and its proper curvature without irregularity.

Perichoroidal Space is a very fine space deep to the sclera, and it contains the fine ciliary nerves passing to the cornea, ciliary body, and iris.

Choroid lies inside the sclera and is the most posterior part of the uvea (see Fig. 2.18).

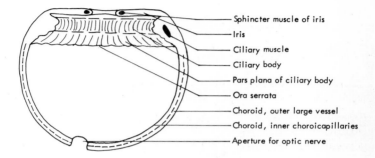

Sphincter muscle of iris
Iris
Ciliary muscle
Ciliary body
Pars plana of ciliary body
Ora serrata
Choroid, outer large vessel
Choroid, inner choroicapillaries
Aperture for optic nerve

Fig. 2.18 Uvea

The choroid is composed mainly of blood vessels (vein and arteries outside and capillaries inside) which supply the nutrition of the outer layers of the retina (especially the rods and cones). These vessels are derived via the short posterior ciliary arteries from the ophthalmic artery and they drain to the venae vorticosae.

The choroid extends from the border of the optic disc to the posterior border of the ciliary body (about 7 mm behind the limbus) at the ora serrata of the retina.

The choroid contains numerous pigment cells, which absorb light and help prevent intraocular scatter of light; the commonest intraocular tumour is melanoma of the choroid.

Ciliary Body is anterior to the choroid and its epithelium forms the ciliary processes, which secrete aqueous into the chamber behind the iris – the posterior chamber (see Fig. 2.20).

The main bulk of the ciliary body is the ciliary muscle, smooth muscle fibres supplied by the 3rd cranial nerve and providing for the function of *accommodation*. The lens of the eye is attached to the ciliary body by the zonule (or suspensory ligament), which relaxes when the ring of ciliary muscle contracts (see Fig. 2.19).

Relaxation of the zonule allows the anterior surface of the lens to become more rounded and therefore increases its focal power, as is required when attending to near objects or reading (accommodation).

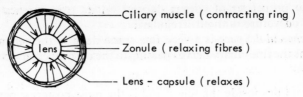

Fig. 2.19 Zonular attachment

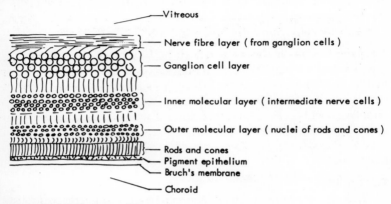

Fig. 2.20 Retinal nerve cell layers

Iris is a thin disc composed of loose spongey connective tissue, within which are contained blood vessels, pigment cells and muscle fibres. The iris root is attached to the anterior border of the ciliary body. It divides the aqueous chamber into a larger anterior chamber and a smaller posterior chamber.

The iris structure consists of three layers:

1. Anterior surface composed of an incomplete epithelium and crypts.
2. Loose connective tissue and blood vessels, with the sphincter muscle near the pupil.
3. Posterior epithelium, which contains most of the pigment cells and the dilator muscle fibres.

Colour of eyes: Brown has pigment in layers 2 and 3.
Blue has pigment in layer 3.
Albino has no pigment and consequent visual defect.

Muscles of Iris:

1. Sphincter pupillae – a ring 1 mm wide near pupil. Constricts pupil in light or near reflexes.
2. Dilator pupillae – fibres radiate from pupil near back of iris. Dilates pupil, as with sympathetic stimulation (fright and flight).

Retina is the innermost layer and part of the central nervous system. It contains the visual cells (rods and cones) which respond to light. Retinal structure consists of layers of nerve cells separated by layers containing the synaptic connections and supported by neurological connective tissue (neuroglia).

The nerve cells are typically found in three layers (see Fig. 2.20).

1. The outer molecular layer consists of visual cells.
2. The inner molecular layer consists of intermediate nerve cells.
3. The ganglion cell layer consists of those cells forming the fibres, which continue from the retina to form the optic nerve.

The blood supply of the retina is from both surfaces, the retina being 'sandwiched' between the choroid outside and the retinal circulation inside. As with the cells of the brain ('grey matter'), the retina has a very high and constant demand for oxygen; the failure of either circulation will result in a hypoxic death of retina cells and consequent partial or complete visual loss.

Ora serrata is the saw-like anterior border of the retina with the ciliary body.

The retina has two special areas:

1. *Optic disc* is where the ganglion nerve fibres of the retina converge (blind spot) and leave the eye as the optic nerve. Here the retinal blood vessels enter the eye (see Fig. 2.21).

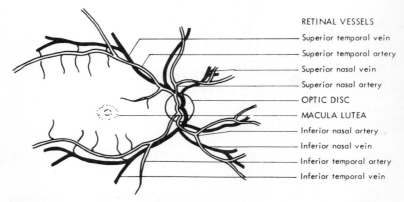

RETINAL VESSELS
Superior temporal vein
Superior temporal artery
Superior nasal vein
Superior nasal artery
OPTIC DISC
MACULA LUTEA
Inferior nasal artery
Inferior nasal vein
Inferior temporal artery
Inferior temporal vein

Fig. 2.21 Ophthalmoscopic view of retina

2. The *macula lutea* (yellow spot) is that part of the retina directed at the object of visual attention, has the highest acuity, and lies on the visual axis which is the line of directed vision passing through the object of visual attention. It contains cones but no rods. Its function is assisted by:

a. Absence of retinal blood vessels anterior to macula.
b. Macular retina is thinned into a depression (the fovea centralis).
c. Each cone has a separate ganglion cell; elsewhere as many as 200 visual cells connect through to each ganglion cell.

Transparent media of the eye comprise the cornea, aqueous, lens and vitreous.

Lens of the eye is formed by the infolding of ectoderm, that layer destined to become the epidermis of the skin. As with the epidermis, the lens-epithelium continues to produce cells throughout life and the lens slowly grows, but also becomes harder (sclerosis). It is a biconvex body posterior to the pupil and iris and is supported within its capsule mainly by the zonule but also by the pupillary area of the iris. Relaxation of the zonule and the resulting increased curvature of the lens allows accommodation of the eye when focusing near objects, but this facility gradually fails when the lens becomes harder with age, usually about 45 years. The lens consists of its elastic capsule, epithelium, cortex and nucleus. It is nourished by the aqueous and has no nerve supply. (See Figure 2.22).

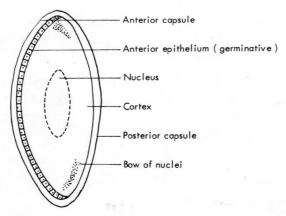

Fig. 2.22 Structure of lens

Aqueous of the eye is a clear fluid secreted by the ciliary epithelium, into the posterior chamber, passes through the pupil, and leaves the eye by the trabecular meshwork of the filtration angle, Canal of Schlemm and aqueous veins (back to the orbital circulation) (Fig. 2.23).
It is a clear fluid, 99 per cent water, with three functions:

1. Pressure of aqueous formation maintains shape of eye.

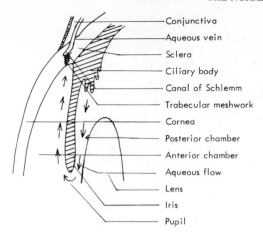

Fig. 2.23 Aqueous circulation

2. Nourishment of lens, and posterior cornea.
3. Transmission of light.

The 1 per cent of dissolved solids includes salts, glucose, urea and Vitamin C. Any interference with aqueous flow or drainage can produce glaucoma, by increasing the aqueous-pressure (normal = 10 to 20 mmHg).

Vitreous is a clear watery jelly filling the posterior segment of the eye from the retina to the back of the lens. With age the vitreous contracts forwards, leaving fluid between it and the retina, and if it adheres to the retina, this may tear with a consequent detachment of the retina. Small opacities in the vitreous are common and may be observed in the field of vision (muscae volitantes or vitreous floaters). Until later life the vitreous is attached by its membrane, the hyaloid membrane to the posterior capsule of the lens. It is nourished by diffusion from the vessels of the retina, choroid and ciliary body.

THE LACRIMAL APPARATUS

The tear-fluid keeps the surface of the cornea and conjunctiva moist, and blinking evenly wets the exposed part of the eye. There is a general motion of the tears from the lateral part of the palpebral fissure below the lacrimal gland towards: (1) the medial canthus where there forms a 'lacrimal lake' draining through (2) the canaliculi to the lacrimal sac, naso-lacrimal duct and nose (see Fig. 2.24).

The naso-lacrimal duct lies in the bony naso-lacrimal canal, which

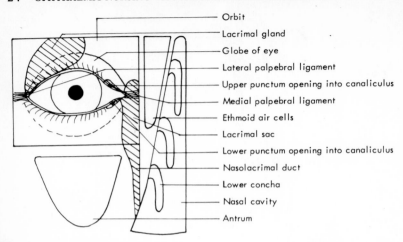

Orbit
Lacrimal gland
Globe of eye
Lateral palpebral ligament
Upper punctum opening into canaliculus
Medial palpebral ligament
Ethmoid air cells
Lacrimal sac
Lower punctum opening into canaliculus
Nasolacrimal duct
Lower concha
Nasal cavity
Antrum

Fig. 2.24 Lacrimal apparatus

opens medial to the antrum and below the inferior concha. Infection can pass up the duct from the nose to cause dacryocystitis (inflammation of the sac) or conjunctivitis (inflammation of the conjunctiva). Epiphora (watering of the eye) can be caused by impaired lacrimal drainage:

1. ectropion (out-turning of the lower eyelid);
2. obstruction of the canaliculi (canaliculostenosis);
3. obstruction of the lacrimal sac or duct (dacryostenosis);

as well as by increased lacrimal secretion as caused by emotion, by trauma, chemical irritants or inflammation.

THE EYELIDS

The eyelids protect the eye from injury and excessive light; blinking helps distribute the tear fluid and to remove dust or fine foreign bodies. The eyelids consist of five layers (see Fig. 2.25).

The blood supply of the eyelid is the terminal branches of the ophthalmic artery, which anastomoses with the angular artery near the nose.

The sensory nerve for the eyelids is the *trigeminal* (5th) nerve; ophthalmic branch (frontal division) to upper eyelid and maxillary to the lower eyelid.

The glands of the eyelid include:

1. The *Meibomian glands* which lie in the tarsal plate and open on to

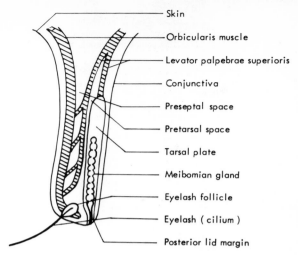

- Skin
- Orbicularis muscle
- Levator palpebrae superioris
- Conjunctiva
- Preseptal space
- Pretarsal space
- Tarsal plate
- Meibomian gland
- Eyelash follicle
- Eyelash (cilium)
- Posterior lid margin

Fig. 2.25 Section of upper eyelid

the posterior lid margin. Their greasy secretion prevents the spillage of water tears and seals the lids during sleep. Infection may often result in chronic swelling of eyelid (*chalazion*).

2. *Glands of Moll* are small sweat glands near root of eyelashes.
3. *Glands of Zeiss* are small sebaceous (sebum-producing) glands also near the root of the eyelashes.

CONJUNCTIVA

The conjunctiva is a thin skin-like membrane joining the eye (at the corneal-limbus junction) to the eyelids. It is firmly attached at the limbus and to the posterior aspect (*tarsal plate*) of the eyelid, but between forms a deep loose fold (*fornix*) to allow for ocular movements (see Fig. 2.26). At the medial end of the palpebral fissure, the *caruncle* (a small fleshy protuberance) represents part of the eyelid separated by development of the lower canaliculus. Between it and the cornea, the semi-lunar fold of conjunctiva represents the vestigial 'third eyelid' (fully developed in birds and cats, etc.). The glands of the conjunctiva consist mainly of many small mucous cells which help to moisten and lubricate, together with some small accessory lacrimal glands (of Krause). Chronic inflammation of the conjunctiva tends to lead to a proliferation of the mucous glands, which may block and form small cysts. The blood supply is from the terminal branches of the ophthalmic artery. Near the limbus the arteries form two layers:

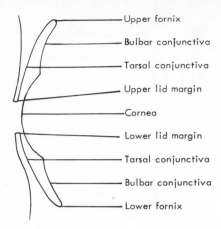

Upper fornix

Bulbar conjunctiva

Tarsal conjunctiva

Upper lid margin

Cornea

Lower lid margin

Tarsal conjunctiva

Bulbar conjunctiva

Lower fornix

Fig. 2.26 Section of conjunctiva

1. Superficial arteries from arteries of eyelid which dilate in *conjunctivitis*.
2. Deep arteries from anterior ciliary arteries which dilate in *iritis*, producing a circum-corneal flush (ciliary flush).
Both layers connect to a limbal arcade of vessels.

EXTRAOCULAR MUSCLES

There are several principal extraocular muscles:

1. The *levator palpabrae superioris* muscle is inserted into the superior border of the tarsal plate of the upper eyelid, which it elevates.
2. The other six are concerned with ocular movement (see Fig. 2.27).

Origins of muscles
1. *Inferior oblique muscle* arises anteriorly from orbital margin lateral to naso lacrimal canal.
2. All other six arise at apex of orbit, mainly from *annulus of Zinn* (Fig. 2.28).

Insertions of muscles
1. *Rectus* muscles insert into the scleral ring 6 to 8 mm behind the limbus (see Fig. 2.15).
2. *Oblique* muscles pass below recti of same prename (superior, inferior) to be inserted behind the equator of the eye.

Function of these six muscles is to move (rotate) the eye about its centre 12 mm behind the cornea.

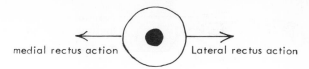

medial rectus action   Lateral rectus action

(a) horizontal muscles

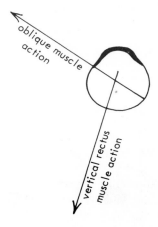

oblique muscle action

vertical rectus muscle action

(b) vertical muscles

Fig. 2.27 Ocular muscle planes

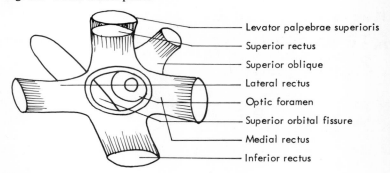

Levator palpebrae superioris

Superior rectus

Superior oblique

Lateral rectus

Optic foramen

Superior orbital fissure

Medial rectus

Inferior rectus

Fig. 2.28 Annulus of Zinn

Single eye movements occur as the muscle acts to move the eye as a lever about its fulcrum, the centre of the eye (see Fig. 2.29).

Types of movement (see Fig. 2.30).
Binocular movement of the eyes may be:
1. Conjugate, when the eyes move equally in the same direction; the muscles paired in this movement are yoke muscles (see Fig. 2.31).

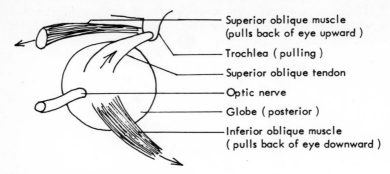

Fig. 2.29 Oblique muscle action

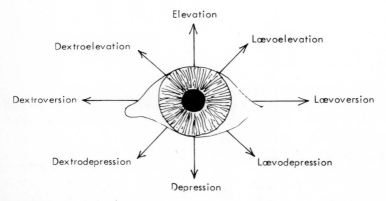

Fig. 2.30 Movements of eye

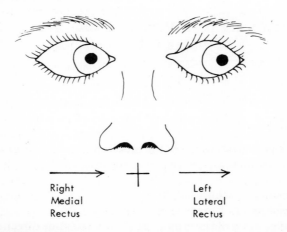

Fig. 2.31 Yoke muscles

2. Disjugate, when the eyes move equally in opposite directions, as when they converge for near vision (see Fig. 2.32).

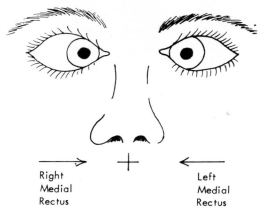

Fig. 2.32 Convergence

Levator palpabrae superioris muscle:
1. Origin – with superior rectus, from annulus of Zinn and apex of orbit; muscles separate anteriorly as levator spreads out to width of eyelid.
2. Insertion into upper eyelid: skin, tarsal plate, fornix of conjunctiva, and into the medial and lateral palpebral ligaments.
3. Nerve supply is partly by the oculomotor (3rd) nerve, and partly by sympathetic nerve fibres. The first controls the voluntary movement of the upper eyelid and the sympathetic controls the involuntary tone of the muscle, which is reduced in sleep and excessive in fear or in *hyperthyroidism* (Grave's disease). The involuntary part of this muscle is known as Müllers muscle.

THE EYE AS A SELF-CONTAINED SYSTEM

The eye has so far been studied as a self-contained system from the point of view of the structure and function of its parts, as in the practice of ophthalmic nursing a detailed knowledge of these parts is essential. The eye is part of the body, but much of the basic knowledge of this body has been gained by a more detailed knowledge of its parts, and particularly the cell, which is the unit for which both life and disease can be defined. It is with the death of its component cells that the body as a whole eventually dies, and it is also within the living cell that most of the pathological and biochemical changes of disease occur. Cells share a common structure (nucleus, cytoplasm, cell membrane, etc.) and, within each individual person, a common genetic inheritance (see Fig. 2.33).

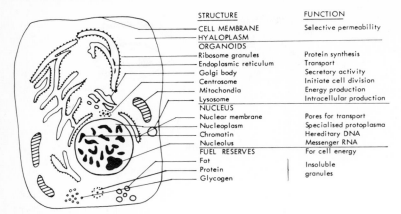

STRUCTURE	FUNCTION
CELL MEMBRANE	Selective permeability
HYALOPLASM	
ORGANOIDS	
Ribosome granules	Protein synthesis
Endoplasmic reticulum	Transport
Golgi body	Secretory activity
Centrosome	Initiate cell division
Mitochondia	Energy production
Lysosome	Intracellular production
NUCLEUS	
Nuclear membrane	Pores for transport
Nucleoplasm	Specialised protoplasma
Chromatin	Hereditary DNA
Nucleolus	Messenger RNA
FUEL RESERVES	For cell energy
Fat	
Protein	Insoluble granules
Glycogen	

Fig. 2.33 Cell structure

The health of each cell is maintained by the constant composition of the extracellular fluid, which in turn depends on adequate circulation containing blood of a composition controlled by other systems such as blood-forming marrow, the gas-exchanging lungs, and the water-and-salt excreting kidneys. These extracellular fluids were defined in the last century by Claude Bernard as an *internal environment*, and nursing may be considered partly as supporting those bodily functions which maintain the constancy of the internal environment.

The aqueous fluid and vitreous body form a large part of the internal environment of the eye. The aqueous is continually replaced by secretion and drainage, and is responsible for the nutrition of the lens: it contains small concentrations of protein, glucose, electrolytes such as sodium, calcium, potassium, and chloride ions, as well as a fairly high concentration of ascorbate (Vitamin C). These substances are derived from the blood supply of the ciliary epithelium, which secretes the aqueous, so that the biochemistry of the aqueous is dependent on the chemistry of the blood as well as the metabolism of the epithelial cells. However, the mechanism of aqueous flow and the resulting intra-ocular pressure can well be studied as a system enclosed by the corneoscleral envelope with a secretic pressure created by the ciliary epithelium (see Fig. 2.34).

In this system the drainage of aqueous at the angle of the anterior chamber is probably passive, but the resistance to aqueous outflow can change and may be controlled by the apertures in the trabecular

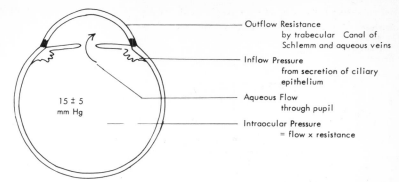

Fig. 2.34 Intraocular pressure

meshwork. In *glaucoma* an increase in resistance to outflow is more usual than an increase in inflow (secretion); the decrease in outflow may reduce the inflow (see Fig. 2.35).

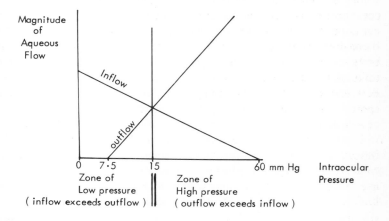

Fig. 2.35 Control of inflow and outflow to regulate pressure

Small increases in volume produce large increases of pressure in this mechanically closed system, and glaucoma is associated with changes to the blood flow through the eye. As the intra-ocular pressure increases above its normal (15 ± 5 mmHg) there is a progressive compression of the vessels, firstly the veins and ultimately the arteries, resulting in ischaemia; this may be compared to the effect on the blood flow of the arm by a sphygmomanometric cuff (see Fig. 2.36).

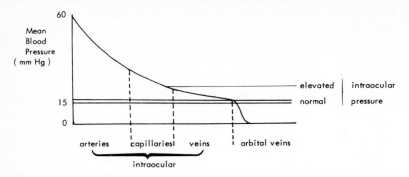

Fig. 2.36 Effect of elevated intraocular pressure compressing veins before capillaries and arteries

THE EYE AS PART OF THE BODY

In geography a detailed knowledge of one's own home town and its hinterland must be balanced by an appropriate knowledge of the whole homeland and the foreign countries with which the town communicates, trades and participates in government. Similarly the eye depends on the whole body for its nutrition, which is conveyed by the blood circulation, and it participates in the government of the body as an important sensory organ, transducing light-modulated information into neurological data. As a part of the body its cells are all derived from the single zygote formed by the union of ovum and sperm. The retinal structure develops from the embryonic neural groove (central nervous system) as an optic vesicle at about the third week after conception. The rest of the eye develops in relation to the retina, which with its optic nerve remains an integral part of the central nervous system. The blood circulation develops to nourish the eye and especially the retina, which, as stated above, has a double blood supply, from both retinal and choroidal vessels. This circulation is dependent on the normal functioning of the heart, lungs, and major blood vessels and the eye may be affected in blood disease (*leukemia, anaemia*), in diseases of the vessel walls (*arteriosclerosis, arteritis*) and in diseases of the circulation (*circulatory shock, heart-failure, embolism*).

The intra-ocular pressure was considered in the previous section as partly dependent on the closed structure of the eye. However, it is also affected by circulatory changes; a failure of the blood supply will reduce aqueous formation and lead to a soft eye (*hypotony*) and an obstruction to the venous channels of the orbit will reduce aqueous outflow and lead to an increase in pressure (*glaucoma*). There is also evidence that the intra-ocular pressure is at least partly controlled by nerve-centres in the base of the brain, but the detailed nerve pathways are not known.

The eye contains within its structure cells representative of most of the tissues which make up the body, for instance:

1. *Epithelial* cells are found on the surface of the cornea and conjunctiva in continuity with the epidermis; the eye can be affected in many skin diseases (*herpes simplex*, dermatitis, allergy, psoriasis, pemphigus).

2. *Connective tissue* fibres are found in the sclera and stroma of the cornea and may be affected in connective tissue disease (rheumatoid diseases, brittle bone disease).

3. *Blood-vascular* tissues are found in two systems; the uvea (iris, ciliary body, and choroid) and the retinal circulation; these are affected in many diseases of the circulation, *diabetes* and inflammations.

4. *Muscle fibres* are found in the pupil muscles, ciliary muscle and the muscles of the orbit; these can be weakened in muscle disease (myasthenia gravis, myopathies) or by diseases affecting the motor nerves supplying the muscles (head injuries, brain tumour, *encephalitis*, neuritis).

5. *Nerve* cells of the central nervous system are found in the retina, which may be affected by neurological disease (*multiple sclerosis*, toxic drugs such as *chloroquine*). Nerves of the peripheral nervous system provide innervation of the muscles (affected in peripheral neuritis) and sensation for the eye and face (affected in shingles, *herpes zoster* ophthalmicus, which is an infection of the trigeminal ganglion and nerves).

The eye is not only complex in its structure, but also in its function, as will now be shown.

THE EYE AS PART OF THE VISUAL SYSTEM

The optics of the eye (see Fig. 2.37). have been compared with the optics of a camera.

It is emphasised that the cornea is the most powerful focusing surface for the eye, whereas the lens allows for a change of focus by its flexible shape. Briefly the comparison can be tabulated:

Quite small variations in the shape and size of the eye produced by normal growth or by disease can displace the optical image forwards (myopia) or backwards (hypermetropia) (see Fig. 2.38).

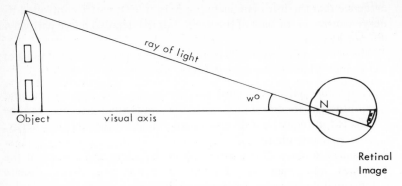

Fig. 2.37 Optics of the eye. Light is refracted by the cornea and lens to form the retinal image, which is encoded by the retina into a neurone pattern of information. The angular size of the object (w°) is the angle subtended at the nodal point of the eye (N).

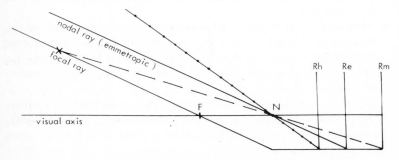

Fig. 2.38 Geometry of myopia and hypermetropia. Focal ray through focus (F) is refracted parallel to visual axis and meets nodal ray at retinal image. Myopic retina (Rm) is posterior to emmetropic (Re) and nodal ray converges to X, far point of accommodation. Hypermetropic retina (Rh) is anterior to emmetropic and its nodal ray is divergent from focal ray.

Table 2.1

	Eye	Camera
Skeleton	Sclera	Box
Black-lining	Pigment	Black paint
Lens system	Cornea + lens	Lens
	Pupil and iris	Iris-diaphragm
Control of light	Adaptation of retina	Change of film-speed
Image (inverted)	On the retina	On the film
Focusing	Altered shape of lens	Altered position of lens

The visual disability of myopia can be corrected by a minus (concave) spectacle lens, which shifts the far image backward to the retina, whereas hypermetropia is corrected by a plus (convex) lens which shifts the optical image forward. Plus lenses are also used in presbyopia, when, in later life, the near (reading) object can only be focused to an image behind the retina.

In astigmatism the degree of myopia or hypermetropia varies according to a direction at right-angles to the visual axis and this can often be corrected by a cylindrical (in contrast to the more usual spherical) lens.

Even when the focusing of the eye is 'perfect' the retinal structure and function is such that it responds to it in a complicated way, producing fine acuity only for the central macular area. Retinal functions can be summarised:

1. *Visual acuity* is the ability to discriminate parts of the image, is related to the fineness of the matrix of visual cells, and falls off rapidly outside the macula. It is measured by tests such as Snellen's non-serif type, Albini's E-test and Sheridan's Stycar.

2. *Colour vision* is also confined to the central retina, is related to the presence of cones, and congenital colour-blindness is inherited as a sex-linked recessive (affecting about 8 per cent men). It can be tested by Ishihara plates, lantern tests, or colour-tint matching.

3. *Dark adaptation* occurs rapidly for the central retina, but more slowly and to a far more sensitive level for the peripheral retina, where there are mainly rods and not cones. It requires specialised equipment for testing (adaptometer) and is often defective in diseases of the retina such as *glaucoma* and *retinitis pigmentosa*.

4. *Peripheral vision* has a low acuity, but the visual field is important for total visual awareness. There is a wide choice of equipment for charting the visual field, but often a fairly useful idea of the field may be gained by facing the patient (confrontation) and checking his field in comparison with one's own using a moving figure or a small round target (white or coloured). Changes in the visual field are extremely important in neurological disease as may be understood when looking at the rest of the visual pathways.

The retina connects by the ganglion cell fibres through the optic nerves, chiasma and optic tracts to the lateral geniculate body, which in turn relays visual information to the visual cortex of the occipital lobes of the cerebrum (see Fig. 2.39).

It will be noted how the nasal fibres (stimulated by light from the temporal field) cross at the chiasma. Lesions of the chiasma (B), will tend to produce bitemporal hemianopia; lesions anterior to the chiasma (A) will affect one visual field only; lesions posterior to the

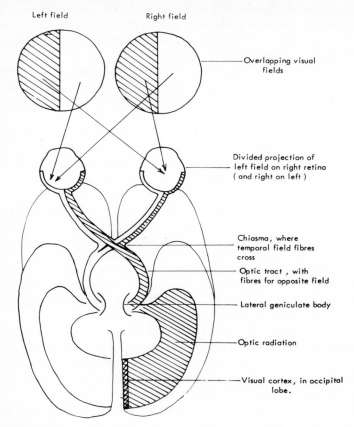

Fig. 2.39 Visual pathway

chiasma (C) will tend to produce a homonymous hemianopia (see **Fig. 2.4**).

These patterns of field loss may be important for locating the disease process. The structure of the visual pathway with the chiasma crossing also form an essential basis for binocular vision.

5. *Binocular vision* is a function whereby the two retinal images are perceived as a single 'fused' image. The disparity of the images forms a basis for stereopsis. Binocular vision is usually defective in squint, and is tested by the orthoptist using the cover test (alternative covering of each eye which is fixating on an object), prism-shift, synoptophore, Titmus stereo test, etc.

The visual function of the two eyes probably only comes together properly at the cerebral cortex.

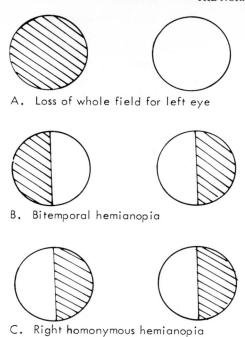

A. Loss of whole field for left eye

B. Bitemporal hemianopia

C. Right homonymous hemianopia

Fig. 2.40 Defects of visual field

PSYCHOLOGICAL ASPECTS OF VISION

Much of the knowledge of the psychology of vision has come from a study of those who have either been born blind or those who have lost their sight later in life, as well as more recent experiments in sensory deprivation (covering the eyes or living for long periods in total darkness). These changes may be summarised:

1. *Sensory.* Those born blind are often fully adapted by using other senses, especially hearing and touch. The aesthetic response to proportion is altered and haptic detail is often more important than overall relations; a square often seems preferred to the rectangular 'golden-section'.

2. *Social.* Communities and language are important to social relations and in modern society the written language is increasingly important. A blind person may compensate by use of Braille, but this will not be easily read by others, and the books are necessarily large and bulky. In reverse the blind person may depend on others to read to him confidential letters, with an implicit loss of privacy. In social

conditions, including hospitals, the blind person needs to be seen as one who cannot always be aware of the presence of that other person, with whom he wants to communicate. In many ways he will continue to be dependent on the goodwill of others, although in childhood maximum independence is to be encouraged.

3. *Occupational.* Many occupations are essentially visual, but may often be adapted for haptic sensation by a blind person. Even so some techniques (e.g. electronics) become increasingly fine and what once could be usefully done by a blind person can no longer. The blind are therefore continually dependent on others for the adaptation of occupations, but they also are able to concentrate well on the job, having reduced visual distraction, and compete well in suitable occupations. The older person may, on becoming blind, be unable to continue work and this itself may lead to severe psychological problems such as exogenous depression.

With hearing, vision extends man's awareness well beyond his own environment. Man's experience of himself as a small element in the cosmos under the stars of the night sky has moulded much of his religious and cultural background as well as inspiring much of his interest in modern science. It is not surprising that as the most visually developed ape, man should feel threatened by eye disease which may deprive him of sight; the ophthalmic nurse should appreciate this and reassure the patient in an informed and sympathetic manner.

3

Ophthalmic nursing practice

Psychophysical aspects
Ophthalmic nursing routines (medical,
surgical)
Ophthalmic nursing planning

PSYCHOPHYSICAL ASPECTS OF OPHTHALMIC NURSING

Efficient nursing care depends on an evaluation of the patient's needs. These needs arise directly from the nature and effects of the disease (pain, immobility, blindness, etc.) and also from the effects of increased socio-economic dependence and insecurity. Traditionally the doctor has had, and continues to have, a primary responsibility for patient care, but improved standards of nurse education have expanded the role of nursing care and the responsibility of the nurse. The nurse must not only carry out the treatment programmes prescribed by the doctor, but must monitor their effects and be able to initiate changes in the care of the patient, with the further help of the doctor as required. The nurse often communicates with the patient at a more informal and personal level than does the doctor and in these circumstances the patient can impart information important to the complete evaluation of the patient's needs. This type of information requires to be documented in a confidential and systematic way, as will be described in the final section of this chapter (p. 51).

The clinical methods used in the evaluation of a patient's disease underwent a revolutionary change towards the end of the eighteenth century. The establishment of post mortem examination as routine for patients dying in hospital led not only to a greater concern for accurate diagnosis, but also to an increasing correlation of the pathological findings with the associated symptoms and signs found in the clinic. In eye disease it is not often that the eye is removed and therefore available for pathological examination; nevertheless it is still important to recognise those clinical clues presented by the patient and relate them to the underlying patterns of disease. These clues arise from the symptoms (subjective experience of patient) and the signs (objective examination by nurse), which are conveniently separated but may also coincide (as when the patient notices a red eye, an eyelid tumour or a *ptosis* in a mirror and he examines it objectively more or less as the doctor and nurse do.

In science and technology objective knowledge has generally come to be preferred to the subjective experience of the individual. Medical diagnosis, concerned with the diseased state of individuals, relies more or less equally on both the subjective symptoms, which usually bring the patient to his doctor, and the more objective signs of disease revealed by the clinical examination of the patient. In any disease the balance may vary between a total emphasis on symptoms, as in *migraine*, or their total absence, as in presymptomic simple *glaucoma*. In this section consideration is given to those aspects of disease associated with common ophthalmological symptoms: pain and headache, visual disturbances, and mirror-symptoms (abnormalities noted by the patient in a mirror).

Some of the information given in this chapter is tentative, but the emphasis is on the principles of good nursing practice, which is essential in ophthalmic nursing. The aim is the co-ordination of good nursing methods with a simple and accurate record, which will ensure accurate communication between all those responsible for the patient's recovery.

1. Ophthalmological pain

The division of pain into superficial and deep reflects both a difference in character as well as in the anatomical location of the nerve receptors arranged at various levels in the skin and conjunctiva and those in the deeper structures such as the iris and the orbit.

These may be:

a. Local pricking or gritty sensation arising from the conjunctiva or cornea (which is even more sensitive).

b. More generalised aching sensation, arising from the iris or ciliary body, often referred to the upper and lower eyelid and eyebrow.

c. Diffuse aching of both eyes arising with ocular fatigue, small *refractive errors* or latent *squint*.

d. Deep orbital aching pain increasing on movement of the eyes as in inflammation of the orbit or optic nerve.

e. *Photophobia* (photalgia) is an intense pain associated with *blepharospasm* and produced by light; it is often found with keratitis or other corneal diseases.

f. Intermittent or periodic pain is characteristic of some diseases such as *migraine*, some types of acute *glaucoma*, and recurrent corneal abrasion.

g. Diffuse facial pain including the eye may be a symptom of disease outside the orbit, such as *sinusitis* or *cerebral aneurysm*.

2. Visual disturbances

The complexity of the visual process is matched by the very many different visual symptoms and disturbances. The disturbances are basically optical, when they are due to loss of transparency in the media of the eye, or neurological, when they are due to disease of the retina or visual pathways of the rest of the central nervous system.

a. Distorted visual images may be caused by opacities of the vitreous (if near the retina) or by displacement of the retina, as with retinal elevation or shallow *detachments*.

b. Loss of vision may be complete as with a total vitreous haemorrhage or mature *cataract*, although light should be perceived, which is not the case with complete *atrophy* of the optic nerve.

c. Loss of vision may be partial. A blurring is usual with *refractive errors* or immature *cataract*. Patchy loss in the form of blind spots (*scotomata*) or loss of the visual field occurs with diseases of the retina or visual pathways up to the level of the occipital (visual) cortex.

d. Acute loss of vision occurring in minutes or at most a few hours is likely to be due to an acute obstruction of a retinal blood supply or a blood vessel supplying part of the visual pathway, or it may be due to *glaucoma*.

e. Double vision (*diplopia*) is characteristic of *squint*, although in children suppression or alternation of the visual images usually prevents diplopia. One-eyed (monocular) diplopia may occur when the media prismatically split the light (as in early cataract, or with a dislocated or subluxated lens).

3. Mirror symptoms

Since most of us see our eyes in the mirror several times a day, it is common for patients to have noticed changes in or around their eyes.

a. A red eye is an important finding and may be due to inflammation (*conjunctivitis*, *iritis*) in which pain is also usual; or to *glaucoma* or *subconjunctival haemorrhage*. The distribution of the redness may help in diagnosis (see Fig. 3.1).

b. Spots on the eye may be on the conjunctiva (yellow *pinguecula*, brown *melanoma*, red conjunctival haemorrhage), on the cornea (*pterygium*, corneal scar) or iris (brown *melanoma*).

c. Lumps (or tumours) on the eyelid may be benign warts and cysts or the more malignant *rodent ulcer* or *epithelioma*; a swelling on the side of the nose may be due to inflammation or obstruction of the lacrimal sac.

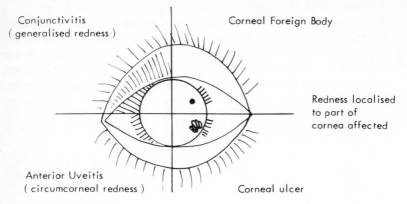

Conjunctivitis
(generalised redness)

Corneal Foreign Body

Redness localised
to part of
cornea affected

Anterior Uveitis
(circumcorneal redness)

Corneal ulcer

Fig. 3.1 The red eye

d. Pus or mucus may be noted, often as a bead near the caruncle; it usually signifies the presence of infection.

e. Crusting of the eyelashes occurs in *blepharitis* and *conjunctivitis* and usually represents dried pus. Loss of eyelashes (madarosis) may occur with *blepharitis* and also in *anaemia*, malnutrition and *myxoedema*.

f. Distortion of the eyelids (*entropion* = turning in; or *ectropion* = turning out) caused by inflammation, swelling or scarring.

An awareness of the relationship of symptoms to disease will help the nurse to ask the patient the most appropriate questions about his condition and will also enable the nurse to appreciate the way in which various eye diseases handicap the patient's social and working life.

OPHTHALMIC NURSING ROUTINES

The separation of medicine and surgery was convenient in mediaeval times when surgeons were non-medical carpenters and the consultant physicians directed patients to either apothecaries for treatment by drugs, or to the surgeon for operation. The medical treatment was mostly safe but usually ineffectual; surgery, even when effectual, was extremely hazardous. Modern ophthalmology has fused these two aspects of treatment within one speciality, but it is still useful to consider their differences; the medical, or non-operative, from the surgical, in which there must be an emphasis on asepsis and the control of infection, the care and preparation of delicate surgical instruments, and the nursing of a patient through the pre- and postoperative periods, including rehabilitation.

Nurses often see a patient as a child rather than as a person with a family; thinking of the patient in relation to his family helps in thinking of him as a person. Nurses cannot appreciate problems they know nothing about, so knowledge increases appreciation. Nurse–patient relationships are two-way; the patient can teach the nurse as well as the nurse help the patient. Nurses need to explore patients' attitudes and behaviour and to question their own role as nurses to serve the patients' needs. Discussion with other members of the health team enlarges our understanding of people and of our interdependence on one another.

Nursing routines will need to change with circumstances and the availability of materials and drugs for treatment, but the principles common to all routines may be summarised:

1. *Purpose and reason* for each routine must be kept clear in order to prevent it degenerating into a superfluous ritual.

2. *Explanation* of the routine to the patient is needed to reassure the patient and also to establish a rapport of communication.

3. *Listing* the routine into a sequence will produce a recognisable procedure, so that, by habit, essential items (e.g. the identification of drugs, dosage, and side) will not be easily omitted. In most cases it is possible to impose a logical sequence on these procedures (generally passing from the subjective towards the objective elements) and this will make it easier for remembering. Avoid cliché and unnecessary jargon which tend to mislead and interfere with communication

In the following section examples of these routines will be described, but it is essential that the student gains experience in constructing similar routines suitable for local facilities. It will be seen that these routines contain elements (e.g. visual acuity, eversion of eyelid) which can be referred to in later chapters, and the page references will be found in the listings.

MEDICAL NURSING ROUTINES

A. Causalty reception and examination

Listing of Routines	Page	Purpose of each element
Room:	67	
Size		Sufficient for equipment and circulation.
Appearance		Clean, good repair, and tidy.
Illumination		Good general illumination as well as focal.
Equipment		Adequate for listed routines.
Storage		Conveniently placed and security as needed.
Desk		Adequate size and conveniently placed for speaking to patient.

Listing of Routines	Page	Purpose of each element
Examination chair		Firm, with headrest, reclining, comfortable.
Couch		Firm, comfortable, adjusting headrest.
Documentation	76	Standard form with numerical identification as well as by patient's name and address; space for both nurse's and doctor's notes; ordered spaces for history, visual acuity, examination, diagnosis, treatment, disposal.
Reception of Patient:	67	
Welcoming remarks		Essential to establish rapport and confidence.
Enquire cause of visit		Assists rapport and identifies problem.
Document details		Name, address, age, sex, employer, occupation, etc.
History:	75	
Symptoms (Sx)		List recent and existing eye symptoms in sequence with any causes apparent to the patient.
Past history		Previous injuries and other eye diseases.
Employment – details		Details of work, especially at time of injury.
Examinations:	77	
Visual acuity		Essential unless very urgent treatment needed.
General appearance		May suggest other injuries, concussion,
Face		etc.
Eyelids		
Conjunctiva		Examination of these structures in a logical order
Cornea		and comparison with the other eye (when
Anterior Chamber		uninjured) is essential if signs of injury
Iris		(haemorrhage, swelling, lacerations,
Pupil		deformity, etc.) are not to be missed.
Diagnosis	73	
		Essential to summarise type of injury and its anatomical location. Diagnosis should explain symptoms and degree of visual loss; doctor must be informed.
Treatment	81	Essential to detail both treatments performed (e.g. removal of foreign body) as well as that dispensed for patient's use.
Explanation		Patient needs to know nature and extent of injury as well as how to use the treatment.
Disposal procedure		Decide on whether patient needs immediate medical or surgical attention or needs review later. Book appointment if necessary.

B. Outpatient reception and care

Listing of Routines	Page	Purpose of each element
Rooms:	83, 89	
Size		Adequate for functions performed.
Number		Adequate for various tasks and privacy.
Communication		Relationship between rooms and corridors for patient-movement and control; visual as well as telephone communication.
Organisation	90	Relationships between staff and with paramedical staff (e.g. records, pharmacy, orthoptics).

Listing of Routines	*Page*	*Purpose of each element*
Equipment	91	As needed by nurses and doctors for listed functions.
Storage	150, 178	Adequate in size, location, and security.
Furniture		Adequate for purpose, comfortable and safe.
Documentation	55	Standard forms with numerical identification as well as name and address; proper space for notes; check part within nurse's responsibility; (e.g. visual acuity, blood pressure and urine-testing). Check changes of address and of doctor, etc.
Reception:	90, 112	Assess relationship to records department and staff.
Introduction		Ensure that patient entering the outpatient area knows purpose of his visit, has appointment and documents.
Regulation of patients		Eye-outpatients usually has many doctors with a complex system of queues; assess pattern of service for each patient and direct accordingly; assess premedical testing required (visual acuity, blood pressure, urine, etc.)
Regulation of waiting		Patients' confidence eroded by excessive waiting; check on excess waiting and seek and give explanation; direct to different queue if appropriate.
Premedical testing		Visual acuity as standard check on visual function; without (s) and with (c) glasses, blood pressure as an indicator of vascular disease in older patients.
		Urine testing for renal disease and diabetes.
		Applanation tonometry as indicator of glaucoma, field if pressure increased.
Introduction to doctor	91	Identify patient by name and corresponding documents. Introduce to doctor with usual common courtesy.
Doctor's equipment		Maintain sufficient communication with clinical areas to supply doctor's needs in the way of equipment, forms, communication, stationery, drugs, dressings, etc.
Doctor's diagnosis and assessment		Check clinical decisions with doctor and notes so that patient may be referred for requested investigations, treatment and further appointments.
Patient's disposal		Explain investigations and aspects of treatment as requested by patient; ensure patient's movement to special clinics, treatment area, or exit via appointment desk.

SURGICAL NURSING ROUTINES

C. Surgical ward reception

Listing of Routines	*Page*	*Purpose of each element*
Rooms:	131	
Size		Adequate wards for beds and circulation space,

Listing of Routines	*Page*	*Purpose of each element*
		day room accommodation, office and treatment area.
Appearance		Clean and comfortable; cheerful not bleak.
Equipment		Adequate for preparation and continued care of patient.
Storage		Sufficient for supplies, patients, and secure.
Toilets and washrooms		Hygienic and suitable for handicapped patients, correct heights, non-slip floor, alternative of shower or bath, electrically safe.
Sluice		For cleaning and storing of equipment.
Reception:	134	
Location		Comfortable and relaxed.
Documentation		Establish rapport with patient, ensure accuracy of patient's details on notes, diagnosis, and prescribed surgery against the admissions-list.
Psychological		Reassure patient about nature and need for surgery; confident within nurse's experience of surgery.
Socio-economic		Assess disruption to patient and his family due to hospital admission; check economic shortfall, national insurance, etc.
Family		Speak to relations as needed, explain visiting times (note difficulties), and times to telephone.
History:	113	
Symptoms		Review patient's symptoms and any change since his outpatient assessment.
Physiology		Check patient's normal physiological functions such as diet, appetite, bowels, micturition, and sleep.
General health		Ask for any non-ocular disease, especially other treatments which need continuing.
Past history		Ask for any past history of serious disease.
Diagnosis		Check patient's knowledge and understanding of his own diagnosis.
Laterality		Check side of diagnosis and of prescribed operation. Lack of this has led to serious legal action for 'wrong-operation'.
Identify patient and side		Check notes again, complete identity bracelet and fix to patient's wrist or ankle.
Consent form		Check consent form and complete ready for patient's and doctor's signatures.
Examination:	140	
Visual acuity		Visual function assessed before all operations and recorded.
Patient comfortable		Use chair with headrest or couch as needed.
External examination		Examine patient, especially for evidence of infection (pimples, rashes, dermatitis, blepharitis), and allergies.
Culture swab		Pre-operative cultures from conjunctival sac are sometimes required before intraocular surgery.
Lacrimal sac washout		Note evidence of blocked duct and type of regurgitation (mucous or purulent).
Urine testing		For glucose and protein.

Listing of Routines	Page	Purpose of each element
Doctor's examination		Doctor will examine patient before prescribing pre-operative medication; requires stethoscope, sphygmomanometer and ophthalmoscope.
Explanation		Complete explanation to patient of ward routines, facilities, visiting parson, etc. Also need for regular time-tabling, likely time of operation, basic needs of hygiene and use of sterile procedures before and after surgery. Patients are encouraged not to smoke as apart from damage to health, they may ignite the eye-pad, and post-operative coughing may cause damage to the eye.

D. Basic eye dressing (2 nurses)

Equipment:
Trolley (cleaned with soap and water)
Top shelf
Working surface clear.
Bottom shelf – first cleaned with Alcowipe.
1 sterile eye dressing pack containing: 1 gallipot
Cotton wool swabs
1 sterile hand towel
1 extra hand towel

Eye pad(s)
Patient's case sheet or treatment sheet
Drops or ointment (as ordered)
Dermiclear or Micropore tape } surfaces
Sachets or bottle of normal saline } wiped
Sterilised sodium chloride 0·9% } with
Scissors } Alcowipe
Eye torch }
Alcowipe
2 gowns
2 masks
Sterile glass rods (if required)

Procedure:

First nurse	Second nurse	Method	Purpose of each element
1. Explain the procedure to patient			To gain co-operation
2. Close windows, if necessary			To prevent draughts
3. Wash hands	Wash hands	Under running water and dry on clean paper towel	Cleanliness

First nurse	Second nurse	Method	Purpose of each element
4. Put on mask, tying all tapes	Put on mask tying all tapes		Aseptic technique
5. Clean trolley shelves and rails		Using Alcowipe	Cleanliness
6. Clean lotion bottles/sachets and unsterile dressing scissors and torch. Place on lower shelf		Using same Alcowipe unless it has become dry	Cleanliness
7. Collect basic dressing packs and any further supplementary packs; treatment sheet, micropore tape and Alcowipe, and treatment. Check expiry dates and banding of autoclave tape.		Place on lower shelf of trolley	Adequate supply of materials; ensuring sterility of packs
8. Take completed trolley to bedside chair		Position trolley to patients affected side	Facilitates smooth dressing technique
9. a. Place patient in comfortable position		Sitting or lying in bed with head well supported	Comfort for patient and ease for nurse
	b. Wash hands	Under running water and dry on clean paper towel	Cleanliness
10.	a. Open outside bag of pack and empty contents on top of trolley	Touching only the outer bag, avoid contact between it and the top of the trolley and ensure that outer hand towel of pack is uppermost	Cleanliness
	b. Attach outer bag of pack to lower rail of trolley	Tape to side of trolley nearest to patient	To receive soiled dressing.
c. Wash hands and forearms		Using soap and water and sterile nailbrush	Cleanliness
d. Dry hands and forearms		Using the outer sterile towel from pack and drying from fingertips towards elbows	Asepsis

First nurse	Second nurse	Method	Purpose of each element
11. Open pack		Touching only the corners of 2nd towel and avoid contact with trolley	Asepsis
12.	Pour saline into gallipot	Check label with clean nurse and pour from a suitable height ensuring that bottle/sachet does not touch the gallipot	Sterility
13.	Remove existing dressing	By holding skin of forehead and cheek whilst removing the tape	Prevents hurting the patient and thus squeezing the eye
14.	Show to clean nurse before discarding		To note whether any discharge/
15.	a. Wash hands	Under running water and dry on clean paper towel	Cleanliness
b. Place 2nd sterile hand towel/paper cap around/on head. Ask patient to keep eyes closed		By covering hair tucking ends under the patient's head	Helps to steady the patient's head and if necessary, nurse can place hand on paper towel
16. Swab patient's eyelids, using the saline		Use left hand to pick up and moisten swabs, and transfer to the right hand for swabbing. Swab from inner canthus outwards, using each swab once only. Discard into paper bag attached to trolley	Any discharge is thus moved away from the punctum and not pushed down it
17. Ask patient to open both eyes and observe the operated/affected eye in detail	Hold pen torch for observation	By directing light on to unaffected eye first and then into affected eye	Comfort of patient
18. Check treatment with second nurse and treatment sheet	Drops: 1. Open 'Minim' container 2. Open pipette container	Empty on to dressing field	Sterility

First nurse	Second nurse	Method	Purpose of each element
	Ointment: 1. Remove cap and hand tube to clean nurse 2. Open pack	Empty on to dressing field	Sterility
19. Instil treatment. Warn patient that it is cold and may sting		*Drops* 1. Ask patient to look up and gently holding down the lower lid, so that a trough is formed, instil one drop and discard 'Minim'. By directing drop into lower fornix, avoiding globe or lid; or 2. Using pipette withdraw a little fluid from bottle. Instil as above and discard the pipette	Less sensitivity of conjunctiva than cornea
		Ointment 1. Ask patient to look up and gently holding down lower lid apply a little ointment from container-tube between lower lid and globe. Avoid touching lid or globe with nozzle of tube; or	Well formed by lower lid and globe holds ointment long enough for absorption
		2. Ask patient to look up, hold down lower lid and gently place ointment between lower lid and globe using sterile glass rod. Discard rod.	Sterility
20. *If necessary*	a. Open pad pack	Empty contents on to dressing field	
b. Ask patient to close eye and apply pad at a slight angle. Hold with micropore tape	Cut off strip of Micropore tape of suitable length	Avoid touching inner surface	Sterility

First nurse	Second nurse	Method	Purpose of each element
21. Apply cartella shield		In same manner as pad	Added protection of globe
22. Remove paper towel from head and ensure that patient is comfortable			
23. Wash hands	Wash hands	Under running water and dry	Cleanliness
24. Dispose of equipment			
25. Sign treatment sheet			Permanent record of treatment

OPHTHALMIC NURSING PLANNING

The planning of nursing care must be based on experience gained in the clinical area as well as reading and study. An adequate system of nurse-care documentation is needed, and many attempts are being made to improve this, mainly through the use of a 'Kardex' system and through a more systematic record of treatments as they are given. There is now a trend towards the use of problem-orientated nursing notes (see Bibliography) based on the methods of Weed. This approach does provide a syntax within which the information can be co-ordinated and a brief description will therefore follow:

Problem-orientated nursing records (POR)

Principles of record:

1. Each entry must relate to a stated problem and be dated (and signed or initialled).
2. Sources of data and basis for decisions are made explicit.
3. Any change in patient's condition is recorded by a progress note.
4. A progress note has a syntax: Subjective information (symptoms), Objective information (examination or observation), Assessment of condition, and Plan to act on the assessment. This syntax may be remembered by the letters **S O A P**.
5. Any change of plan is documented with the reasons for this change.
6. Treatment is monitored and any lack of response to treatment or allergy recorded and new assessment then made.
7. The initial patient-problems arise from the data as given by patient to doctor and nurse and will include medical, social, environmental and economic factors. These often interrelate as with, for example,

smoking, bronchitis, frequent absence from work, and complication after cataract surgery (due to coughing).

8. The planning of medical and nursing care will be based on the documented assessment of the patient's problems arising from the data and diagnosis.

The use of this syntax can be illustrated by an example:

Nurse-care record – patient for lens-extraction

NURSING CARE HISTORY

Patient's Name: Florence Smith   Hospital No. 78/101
Address: 105 High Street
                  Dudding   Date of birth 14.10.1901

Name of admitting nurse: Mary Duke
Admission diagnosis: R and L cataract for surgery

Subjective data

Problem list

1. Vision getting worse last eighteen months; dazzled in sunlight. Glasses no help. Left worse.
2. Eye waters in cold and in wind. Not sore. No pain.

General information

Previous hospital experience: hysterectomy – 1948.

Previous experience in this hospital: attending since 1974 with declining vision, but glasses corrected until last year.

General health: – pain – no.

treatment by G.P.: sleeping tablets and other medication (unknown).

Domestic activity: housework, cooks for self, lives alone, shopping by daughter-in-law, enjoys knitting.

Visitors: son, Michael Smith – telephone 4305.

Expectation of admission – improved vision after operation.

Daily habits

		Time	*Usual food*
a. Meals:	Breakfast	0800	Tea, toast, jam
	Lunch	1300	Sandwich, tea
	Dinner	1800	Meat, vegetables, dessert
	Snacks	1100	Coffee, biscuits
b. Food dislikes:	fatty foods		
c. Allergies:	none		
d. Usual drinks:	tea, coffee with milk, cocoa		

e. Sleep: well with tablet 2300 to 0715
                          Position – supine with two pillows
                                    Blankets – 3
                                    Window – open
f. Hygiene: Bath – weekly (helped by daughter-in-law)
                          Teeth – dentures
                          Elimination – bladder – control normal
                                    bowels – ×1 daily

Patient's questions

1. When can visitors come to see me?
2. How long will I be in hospital?
3. How soon after the operation will I see?

Objective data

1. General state

a. Placid lady, slightly obese.
b. Does not seem to understand much about eye condition, but
   confident in treatment.

2. Examination (pre-surgical)

VA R s 3/60   R c 6/60
      L s 1/60   L c 2/60
Condition: face, lids, conjunctiva all normal
           white eyes with miotic pupils
           no sign of infection

Assessment	Problem	Therapy
Diagnosis:	Cataract	Surgery
Nursing:	Presurgery	Culture (if required by surgeon)
		Sac-washout
		Clip eyelashes (if required by surgeon)
		Identify – side
		Identify – patient
Doctor's examination		Check drugs
		Premedication
		Sedatives
		Consent to operate signed

Assessment	Problem	Solution
Social:	Lives alone	Speak to son
		Speak to social worker
Occupational:	Looks after self	Speak to social worker (for meals-on-wheels, etc.)
Daily activity:	Enjoys knitting	Arrange with occupational-therapist.
Other:	Poor understanding of condition	Explain to patient, or ask doctor to.

(Documentation would continue after this with daily progress notes.)

This type of documentation is an individualisation of the principles described in this chapter. As nursing is so much concerned with individual care, it is important that this type of documentation should be clear and accurate and while including many details, should not become so overloaded as not to be easily read and understood by other nurses, who will, when on duty, take over the responsibility for the patient and may need to act on the information and assessments. There is so much that can be documented that the more experienced nurse will usefully develop an abbreviated style, concentrating on the most important aspects of the patient's care. Experience does create a hierachy of nursing values, in which the patient's immediate physiological survival is obviously more urgent that the long-term convalescence and social rehabilitation. Nevertheless, to concentrate on the short-term nursing problems without planning for the long-term is not good nursing and may lead to so many problems after discharge home that the patient requires early readmission. For example the patient considered above will need cataract-spectacles following operation and unless these are available and are ordered sufficiently early, rehabilitation will be delayed.

Following admission, progress notes on the patient's condition should be regularly documented. Inpatient progress notes should be kept on a regular basis, especially following surgery, and these may follow the **S O A P** syntax, e.g.:

S Patient complains of aching eye
O Nurse notes cornea hazy and cloudy anterior chamber
A Complication affecting anterior segment, query infection
P₁ Duty doctor notified – confirms hypopyon infection
P₂ Doctor plan

    a. Conjunctival swab for culture.
    b. Syringe lacrimal sacs.
    c. Therapy – see treatment chart.

The use of problem-orientated notes has spread since Weed's publication in 1968 (see Bibliography), but the structure of nursing records has not been finally determined and is still developing. Some of the stationery used in one ophthalmic hospital is depicted in Figs 3.2 to 3.6, but the same stationery is often used in various ways and it is the way in which the doctors and nurses determine the record that reflects its quality. The record is a tool that both guides the care of the patient and also teaches those that care for the patient. The essential

SURGEON **Mr. Woodhouse**

SURNAME/FAMILY NAME	CHRISTIAN/GIVEN NAMES	UNIT No.
		DATE
ADDRESS		TELEPHONE No.
		M.S.W.
OCCUPATION/SCHOOL	GENERAL PRACTITIONER (Full name)	AGE
PLACE OF WORK		D.O.B.

DIAGNOSIS	OPERATION
1._____	
2._____	
3._____	
4._____	

R.V.   APPOINTMENT

L.V.

DATE	CERT		TREATMENT

E 43

Fig. 3.2 Record document – front (W.AHA)

syntax of the record is the listing of the clinical problems and the treatments carried out as solutions to the problems; it is in the recognition of the further problems that occur either by the failure of a proposed solution or by the progress of the disease that a wider teaching experience will occur. The continued cycle of the patient's problems and the applied solutions provide a clinical *dialectic*.

Language of the nursing record

So far the nursing record has been considered in terms of statements

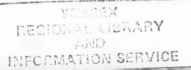

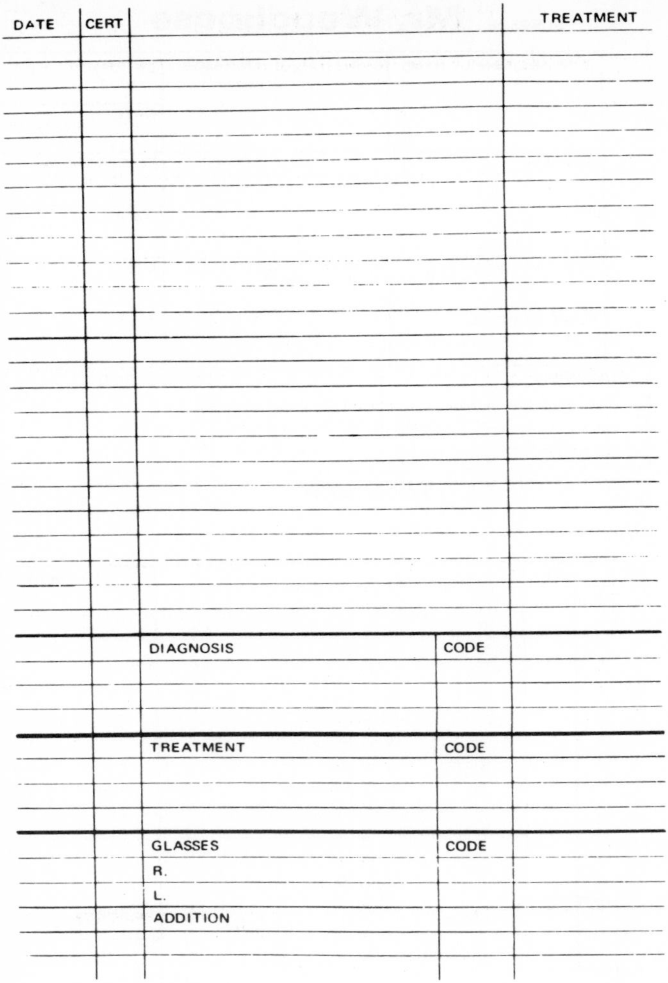

DATE	CERT		TREATMENT
		DIAGNOSIS	CODE
		TREATMENT	CODE
		GLASSES	CODE
		R.	
		L.	
		ADDITION	

Fig. 3.3 Record document – back (W.AHA)

made in a technical prose with problem-orientated syntax. There are also aspects of the report which are of a quantitative or topographical nature and these will require a numerical or pictorial record.

1. *Numerals* have been used in different forms to express various concepts of quantity. Whole numbers (integers) can be used to enumerate entities such as people, cells and limbs. The same numerals can be formed into fractions or be decimalised in order to form a scale of values, as used for drug dosages or on a thermometer

TRAUMA CARD

SURNAME	CHRISTIAN NAMES	UNIT No
		DATE

HISTORY :

Date and time of injury :

Date and time of examination :

Place or Address of factory where injured :

Operation or employment at time of injury :

Machine or tool in use —if any :

Source of injury (e.g. f.b., chemical, toxic substance)
and its composition :

Protection in use at time :

Previous condition of eyes (if known) :

Examination :

Area of injury :   **Type of contamination :**

Details :—

Right   Left

Face
Orbit
Lids
Canaliculi
Conjunctivo-Scleral
Cornea
A.C. (Depth)
Pupil and Reaction
Iris
Lens
Vitreous
Fundus

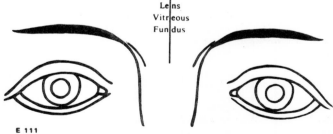

E 111

Fig. 3.4 Trauma record (W.AHA)

scale. Where measurements are made on both sides of a single value,
e.g. freezing point, negative (−) as well as positive (+) numerals are
needed.

IN-PATIENT TREATMENT CARD

Surname:				First Name	
Consultant		Ward	Age		Reg. No.
Drugs from G.P.					

Contra-Indicated Drugs		Weight

Indicated drugs

Drug	Dose or %	Eye or Route
Signatures (1) M.O.	(2) Pharm.	

Date Time													

Drug	Dose or %	Eye or Route
Signatures (1) M.O.	(2) Pharm.	

Date Time													

Drug	Dose or %	Eye or Route
Signatures (1) M.O.	(2) Pharm.	

Date Time													

Fig. 3.5 Treatment card – front page (W.AHA)

Some nurses are unsure in the use of numbers in clerical records, partly because any measurement seems to be mathematical. Much of this unease may have resulted from the modern fashion for

Weight		Once only, Postoperative & Premedication Drugs	Dose	Dr.	Given by: Sign.
Date	Time				

Date   Drugs to take home

Drug	Dose & directions	Route or eye	No. of days	Pharm. Sig.

E61

Fig. 3.6 Treatment card – end page (W.AHA)

modernising the units of measurement (imperial and apothecary to metric and now to SI), but it should be remembered that all units are arbitrary and their clinical use may require no actual knowledge of the physical nature of the unit; the clinical thermometer was put into use for the diagnosis of fever long before the science of thermodynamics related temperature to the agitated movement of molecules. Numbers do give an accuracy to clinical data, and are used when a clinical method has been agreed, but the unit should also be stated; 37°C is not 37°F.

SI units (International System of Units) restrict the units of physical measurement to those derived from a few single basic units such as metre for length, kilogram for mass and second for time. On this basis, force (or weight) is measured in Newtons (kilograms times acceleration as metres per sec. per sec.) and pressure in Pascals (Newtons per square metre). Temperature is measured in degrees Kelvin (°K) which is an identical unit to degrees Celsius (°C) except that the starting point is absolute zero and therefore the freezing point of water, 0°C, is 273°K. In optics the power of lenses is measured in dioptres (the reciprocal of the focal length in metres, $D = 1/m$) and luminous intensity in Candela (cd). The unit of angle is a radian, but in optics and orthoptics the centrad is more often used (1 centrad = $1/100$ rad = $0.57°$). The usual prefixes are used to increase and decrease a unit's value:

tera	(T)	times	1 000 000 000 000
giga	(G)	times	1 000 000 000
mega	(M)	times	1 000 000
kilo	(K)	times	1 000
milli	(m)	divide	1 000
micro	(μ)	divide	1 000 000
nano	(n)	divide	1 000 000 000
pico	(p)	divide	1 000 000 000 000

These units are being adapted gradually through the policy of metrication and it is likely that they will have been fully adopted by the next decade. Until this occurs it is important that the nurse knows and uses those units accepted in her clinical department.

In ophthalmic nursing, numerals are used widely in the measurement of lenses, the testing of visual acuity and visual fields, and the angular measurement of squints, as well as in the routine charting of temperature, pulse and respiration (TPR charts) and of intraocular pressure (phasing). The quantitative evaluation of visual acuity is an example of their use; although the acuity is basically related to the smallest detectable angular difference, a measurement of angle is not often used. As seen in Fig. 3.7 the size of an image on the retina changes as the object becomes more distant from the eye. It has been found that a normal eye can resolve an angular difference of 1 minute (1/60 degree) or better, and the construction of the visual test type is based on this assumption (Fig. 3.8). Visual acuity depends on

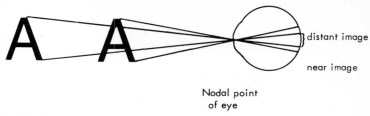

Fig. 3.7 Changing size of retinal image

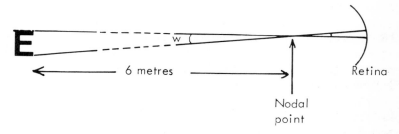

Fig. 3.8 Five elements of E producing retinal image size of 5 minutes of arc (w = 5′)

accurate optics within the eye and also discrimination by the fine sensory elements (rods and cones) of the retina, and the spacing of these allows for an acuity of 1 minute (or somewhat better). For the standard distance of testing at 6 metres, the Snellen's non-serif type is constructed so that the details, as shown, correspond to 1 minute and the whole letter 5 minutes, and such a letter is labelled with a 6 (as it should be able to be seen at 6 metres). The letter labelled 60 is ten times larger and would produce the same angular differences on the retina if viewed at 60 metres, and therefore increases the angular differences to 10 and 50 minutes respectively at 6 metres. Conventionally the acuity is recorded as 6/60 (corresponding to a minimum resolution of 10 minutes), as this preserves in the record the distance of the test-type (on the numerator) and the distance at which the type would normally be read (as the denominator). As a decimal (0·1) this would indicate an acuity of one-tenth or normal, but acuity is not usually recorded this way. The other letters are labelled 36, 24, 18, 12 and 9 down to the normal 6, and are used similarly.

The idea of acuity as an angle is also used in visual field testing, although here the actual measurements are recorded (Fig. 3.9). For instance, if a Bjerrum screen is used at 2 metres, the record of a target as 2/2000 white will indicate a 2 mm white target at 2 metres from the patient.

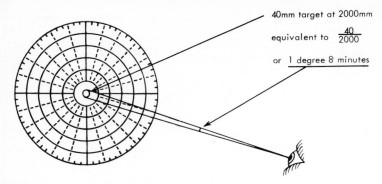

40mm target at 2000mm

equivalent to $\frac{40}{2000}$

or $\underline{1\ \text{degree}\ 8\ \text{minutes}}$

Fig. 3.9 Angle of arc for Bjerrum screen

Since this is a tangent screen:

$2/2000 = 1/1000 = 0 \cdot 001 = 0 \cdot 1$ prism dioptres (or $3 \cdot 43$ minutes)

Again the measurement is angular, but is not expressed as an angle in the clinical records as it is important to retain details regarding the actual size of target and the actual distance from the patient. Surprisingly the illumination of the target and screen, which also affects the test, is rarely recorded.

2. *Diagrams* in the nursing record may be graphical or pictorial.

a. *Graphs* are used when a measurable unit is to be compared with another unit; this latter unit is often time as in the temperature chart. These charts often relate several measurements together, and can visually emphasise related changes. Relevant clinical detail should be added, as in the diurnal record of intraocular pressure (Fig. 3.10); changes of treatment show related changes in pressure.

b. *Pictographs* are used mainly to show the anatomical location of disease and injury (Fig. 3.11) or the location of surgical procedures (Fig. 3.12). They can be very simple, but are still more accurate than many lines of prose description.

Language of assessment and planning

As in medicine and surgery it is a dictum that diagnosis precedes therapy, so also in the problem-orientated record the planning arises logically from the assessment. The assessment will include the clinical diagnosis, but also social, economic, and other personal diagnoses. The complexity of medical diagnosis is perhaps over-emphasised by the long and varied lists of names given to diseases in the ophthalmological textbooks and especially in the official nomenclature of diseases (see Bibliography), the nurse should concentrate on the anatomical location of the disease (as in Chapter 2) and on the

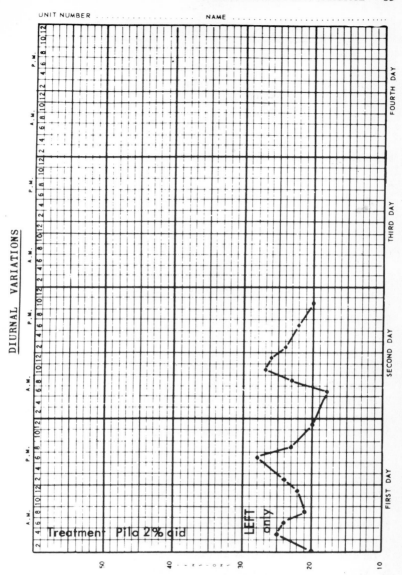

Fig. 3.10 Diurnal record of intraocular pressure (W.AHA)

clinical pathology, as seen through signs and symptoms presented.
  The principal types of clincal pathology are:

1. Circulatory disturbances follow, for instance, *embolism* or

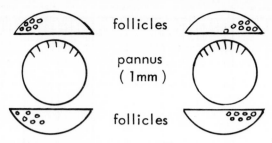

Fig. 3.11 Pictograph of conjunctiva and cornea in trachoma

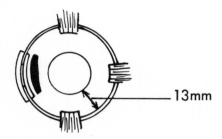

Fig. 3.12 Pictograph of retinal detachment surgery showing distance of strap from limbus and position of plomb beneath disinserted rectus muscle

thrombosis which stop the blood flow to part of the body and this produces hypoxia or gangrene.

2. Degeneration may occur through chronic disease, reduced blood flow, and the replacement of active cells by scar tissue.

3. Dysfunction may occur from a loss of co-ordination, as in a *squint* when the two eyes fail to act together to produce a single binocular perception.

4. Genetic inherited genes producing the chemical messengers which disorganise the normal pattern of development, as with colour-blindness and *albinism*.

5. Inflammation is diagnosed from the classical signs of redness, swelling, pain, and hotness, as with *conjunctivitis* and *iritis*; it may be due to many irritative and other causes as well as infection.

6. Metabolic disease is caused by an upset in the body's chemistry; this is often due to disease of the endocrine glands, as when an over-active thyroid gland produces *Graves' disease* and the associated *exophthalmos*.

7. Nutritional disease results from a lack of specific elements of the diet and is commoner in tropical countries; xerophthalmia is a dry degeneration of the cornea due to lack of Vitamin A.

Anatomical \ Pathological	Circulatory Disorder	Degeneration	Dysfunction	Inflammation
Orbit	thrombosis of orbital veins	atrophy of orbital fat		orbital cellulitis
Lacrimal		Dacryostenosis		Dacryocystitis
Eyelid		Tylosis Cicitrization	Ectropion Entropion	Blepharitis
Conjunctiva	hyperaemia of conjunctiva	Pinguecula		Conjunctivitis
Cornea	pannus	Pterygium		Keratitis
Sclera, Globe		Scleromalacia		Scleritis
Uvea	infarct of choroid	Iris – atrophy		Iritis, uveitis
Pupil		Pupil – atrophy	miosis mydriasis	
Lens		Cataract		
Vitreous	Vitreous haemorrhage	Synchesis	'floaters'	hyalitis
Retina	retinal vessel occlusion	peripheral degeneration	amaurosis	septic retinitis
Optic Nerve		optic atrophy		optic neuritis
Glaucoma	secondary to thrombosis		simple glaucoma	secondary to uveitis

Fig. 3.13 Anatomical and pathological aspects of diagnosis

8. Poisons and other toxic agents are usually diagnosed from the history. The retina is particularly sensitive, and *toxic amblyopia* may occur with tobacco or methylated alcohol, or complicated treatment with drugs such as *chloroquine* and some tranquilisers.
9. Trauma is usually obvious from the history, but the extent may go beyond what is clinically obvious; small puncture wounds of the upper eyelid can penetrate to the frontal lobe of the brain, and *lime burns*, when not treated immediately, can produce progressive vascularisation and opacification of the cornea.

Figure 3.13 shows how the anatomical and pathological features can be related, but even when the pathological condition is not clear, it can be important to relist the main symptoms in the assessment. For example, epiphora (spilling of tears down the face) is almost always indicative of an obstruction of the lacrimal passages, which would therefore need investigation before treatment is planned.

PRIVATE AND IN CONFIDENCE
This should not preclude the availability of information to
authorised persons working with the blind and partially-sighted

Examination for admission to the r

County/Borough of

These details are to be completed before the form is sent to the consultant ophthalmologist

Name of person examined Mr./Mrs./Miss

Address

Date of birth _____ Sex _____ Present occupation

Name and address of general practitioner

The consultant ophthalmologist is requested to complete all sections of this form and return it to

Section A: Examination of the eyes		right eye	left eye
1 Age at onset of condition leading to present visual disability			
2 Age at onset of blindness/partial-sight. (Generally age at which person was unable to follow usual occupation because of visual disability)			
3 Visual Acuity:	(a) unaided		
	(b) with correcting glasses		
	(c) with both eyes together (best vision after correction)		
4 Field of vision: (tick appropriate box)	(a) nil	☐	☐
	(b) less than 10°	☐	☐
	(c) contracted	☐	☐
	(d) central scotoma	☐	☐
	(e) hemianopia	☐	☐
	(f) good	☐	☐
5 (i) Globe as a whole:	(a) tension		
	(b) nystagmus		
	(c) squint		
	(d) proptosis		
	(e) disorganised or absent		
(ii) Individual tissues:	(a) lids		
	(b) conjunctiva		
	(c) cornea		
	(d) sclera		
	(e) iris and ciliary body		
	(f) lens		
	(g) vitreous		
	(h) choroid		
	(i) retina		
	(j) optic nerve		

Fig. 3.14 B.D.8 form

The socio-economic assessment also requires a simple structure based on: income and expenses; the patient's job potential and related occupational stress and hazards; domestic and recreational environment; need for convalescence and rehabilitation. The effect of the clinical condition on the patient's abilities needs assessment, and the BD8 form for blind registration shows this (Fig. 3.14) as it passes from clinical details through diagnosis to prognosis to treatment and occupational recommendations.

4

Casualty ophthalmic nursing

ORGANISATION OF A CASUALTY UNIT

The casualty and the outpatient departments are the two portals of entry for patients to obtain hospital attention. A casualty is a patient without a pre-arranged appointment and will therefore often have acute symptoms due to a non-traumatic eye condition. Nevertheless it is the casualty department which receives the bulk of the trauma patients and in many areas the eye-casualties form up to 20 per cent of the total casualty attendances. In spite of the large numbers of casualties, the departments are usually relatively small; this is because almost all the patients are ambulatory and the majority can be treated in the surgical chair. The large numbers of patients will require an adequate waiting area, but the examination and treatment areas will be related to the number of staff required to service these patients. The department can be considered in terms of its structure and the available equipment, and the plan of a typical casualty department is shown in Fig. 4.1; it is equally important to consider the staffing requirements, the control of patients and patient records, and the relationship of the casualty to the main ophthalmic unit with its casualty ward and to the main sources of injury in the community and industry. As well as contributing to a significant proportion of ward admissions, the ophthalmic casualty often treats as much as a fifth of the total casualty work of an area.

1. Structure of a casualty department (Fig. 4.1)

The entrance to the department should be convenient for pedestrians and near adequate parking. Patients are often visually handicapped and steps should not be incorporated. The reception area is near the entrance and here the patient's details are documented before passing to the waiting area, which should ideally have a separate part for

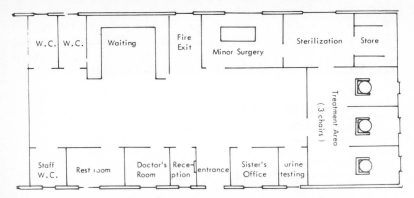

Fig. 4.1 Casualty department (for 20 to 30 thousand per annum; outline plan)

children with some simple and safe play material. The doctor's office and the treatment rooms are all adjacent to the waiting area and the sister's office is centrally placed so that the sister can exercise control over the department and also be easily available. The efficient planning of the department depends vitally on the facilities for transport and communication:

    a. *Transport* involves the ingress of patients through the entrance and reception lobby to the waiting area, and the efficient egress after treatment or admission for inpatient treatment. Easy access is also required for toilets and buffet service. Staff require a separate entrance to the department as well as access to the toilet, buffet and rest facilities. The transport function can also include the efficient supply of equipment (CSSD materials, instruments, and special containers for glass, needles, syringes, etc.), drugs and food and also the disposal of waste, which can include infected materials.
    b. *Communication* within the department will be largely verbal and direct, but signalling devices may be required to show when an examination or treatment room is occupied, vacant or ready for use. Telephone equipment needs to be simple and to provide rapid communication with other hospital departments as well as through the exchange to other hospitals and services.

    An essential aspect of communication is the display of cheerful confidence by the staff within a department which is clean, neat and adequately equipped and furnished.

2. Equipment of an eye casualty department
The equipment of an eye casualty department will include much that is specialised and also fragile and expensive to replace. Storage

cupboards are therefore essential and should be both robust and secure. Clutter from too much floor-standing equipment can be hazardous and may be reduced by wall-mounted cupboards and ceiling-mounted examination lamps. Some equipment merits special attention:

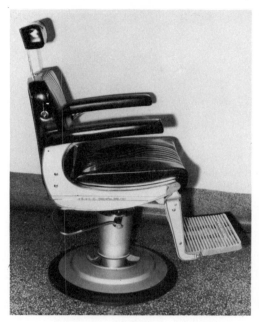

Fig. 4.2 Casualty chair (Clement Clarke)

a. *The examination seat or couch* needs to be firm, secure, and comfortable. The type of seat used in dentistry with a reclining back and headrest is usual (Fig. 4.2). These chairs usually adjust for children, but children are often better examined and treated on a couch and, if necessary, mummified (that is firmly wrapped from neck to toe in a blanket). Any prolonged examination or treatment is preferably carried out with the patient flat on a simple operating table (Fig. 4.3), as the patient is less likely to faint when flat and is more secure even if he does.

b. *The illuminating lamp* for the examination of the eye is extremely important. A concentrated focal beam is required to resolve details of small ocular structures, fine injuries, and corneal foreign bodies. This used to be achieved with a hand-held condensing lens, but today a small ceiling-mounted operating lamp such as that in Fig. 4.4 frees the second hand for securing the patient's head and eyelids

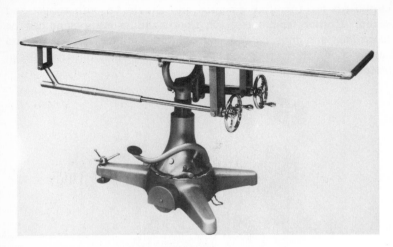

Fig. 4.3 Casualty operating table (Thackray)

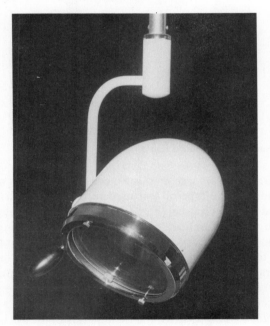

Fig. 4.4 Casualty ceiling light (Hanau, Universal)

while the first holds the operating instrument (such as corneal-f.b. needle). *Skialytic* lamps are to be avoided as the diffusion of the shadows can reduce the operator's perception of detail. Many

patients with eye conditions are sensitive to light (photophobia) and a conveniently placed dimmer control of the thyristor type is useful.
c. *Some magnification* may be required in order to remove fine corneal foreign bodies or for other detailed examination and treatment. A simple magnifying spectacle of the type shown in Fig. 4.5 provides ×3 to ×4 magnification. Higher magnification (×10 to ×20) can be obtained by using the microscope of the slit-lamp, at least one of which should be available in the department.

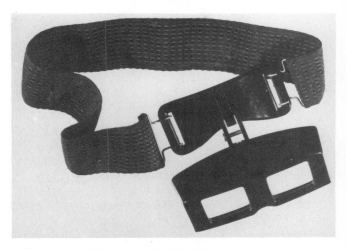

Fig. 4.5 Binomag magnifying spectacles (Keeler)

d. *Visual acuity assessment* of both eyes is essential before any eye treatment as part of the examination of the visual function; lack of a recorded visual acuity exposes the nurse (or doctor) to the legal charge that a future disability could be due to the treatment. The Snellen's non-serif type (Fig. 4.6) is the commonest visual acuity chart and should be well illuminated and placed so that the patient, sitting down, can look towards it at the specified distance of 6 metres (or 3 metres using a mirror). The type is labelled 60, 36, 24, 18, 12, 9, 6, and 5 according to the greatest distance in metres at which a normal eye would easily recognise them. Tested at 6 metres, the acuity should be recorded with the distance as the numerators, e.g.:

VA R$\bar{s}$ $^6/_{60}$ means a '60' type read at 6 metres without glasses by the right eye

R$\bar{c}$ $^6/_9$ means a '9' type read at 6 metres with glasses by the right eye

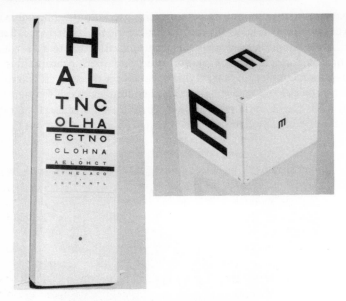

Fig. 4.6 Snellen non-serif type and E-type (Clement Clarke)

Lc̄ CF means the left eye can only count fingers with glasses.

Other abbreviations used are:

HM   for hand movements

PL   for perception of light

NPL for no perception of light

Other tests of visual function should be available:

(i) illiterate tests such as the Stycar (sight test young children and retarded), and E-test (Fig. 4.6).

(ii) Reading-distance charts (N5 to N48).

(iii) Bjerrum screen for testing visual field.

(iv) Amsler charts for testing central field.

(v) Ishihara charts for testing colour perception.

e. *The drugs* available will be the minimum required for casualty treatments and more detail is given in the chapter on drugs. The ocular treatments available will include:

(i) Eye drops (guttae) for examination include topical vital dyes (fluorescin and rose-bengal) and anaesthetic drops (amethocaine, benoxinate).

(ii) Eye drops (guttae) and ointments (oculenta) which contain mydriatics (dilate pupil), miotics (constrict pupil), antibiotics and corticosteroids.

(iii) Tablets such as pain-relieving aspirin, paracetamide and other simple drugs. Diamox (tablets and injection) is used for reducing the intraocular pressure of acute glaucoma, and some systemic antibiotics (penicillin, tetracycline) need to be available.

(iv) Injections available should include:

(a) Soframycin for local subconjunctival injection, and others such as penicillin, colomycin.

(b) Subconjunctival mydricaine (atropine, procaine, adrenalin).

(c) Intramuscular and intravenous diamox and antibiotics.

(v) Eye lotions (collyria) are used mainly for the mechanical washing away of pus or toxic materials; isotonic normal saline is mainly used. Collyria sodium versanate should be available for lime burns.

(f) *Sterile dressings* need to be available in suitably sealed packs. Since injuries often extend beyond the eye to the head and body, a variety of dressings are usually kept in stock such as surgical swabs, strapping, bandages, etc. A supply of protective eyeshields (cartella) are also needed, and dressings and instruments may be grouped in convenient CSSD packs.

OPHTHALMIC ASPECTS OF TRAUMA

Ocular trauma occurs when the eye or its adnexa is subjected to a destructive level of energy; this energy may be mechanical, thermal or chemical.

1. *Mechanical injury* is either to the face and eyelids, to the adnexa, or to the eye itself:

a. Eyelids may be bruised or lacerated by direct trauma and there may be associated fractures or concussive injury to the eye. A large object diffuses the energy over a wider area and tends to result in concussion (bruising) of the tissues, whereas the same energy applied by a small object (pellet or needle point) will break the surface and penetrate with often very little bruising of the tissues. Any laceration of the eyelid needs cleaning and very accurate repair to prevent later deformity caused by cicatrization. Loss of visual acuity indicates involvement of the eye. Diplopia suggests injury to the eye muscles or to the orbit.

b. Laceration of the conjunctiva if small can be left to heal, but usually a suture is required to close the wound. It is important to confirm that the underlying sclera is undamaged.

c. Laceration involving the eye itself, cornea or sclera, usually penetrates through the globe and requires admission to hospital and inpatient surgery. Infection is of immediate danger to the eye, especially if there is a retained foreign body, which may be suggested by the history. Systemic and local antibiotics are needed and an x-ray should always be obtained to confirm or exclude a radiopaque foreign body. *Sympathetic ophthalmia* may develop after a penetrating injury, especially where the ciliary body is affected.

d. Foreign bodies may be deep or superficial, and those on the cornea cause most pain. Intraocular foreign bodies are often painless and may, at least for some time, be symptomless. Foreign bodies penetrate by their *kinetic energy* $(= \frac{1}{2} mv^2)$ so that it is the small high velocity particle, as from a hammer or chisel or grindstone, which most often penetrates.

e. Infection may complicate trauma where there is a laceration or contamination by foreign matter. Conjunctivitis may be due to a foreign body retained under the tarsal plate. A corneal ulcer or abscess may complicate a superficial corneal foreign body and the ulcer itself lead to perforation of the eye and widespread infection (*panophthalmitis*). Intraocular foreign bodies often lead to infection, especially if not removed immediately after injury. All injuries which break the surface of the tissues (laceration, burns) should be treated with antibiotics to prevent infection as far as possible.

2. *Thermal burns* result in a coagulative necrosis of the tissues. The depth and severity of the burn is proportional to the temperature of the causal substance, and this may often be gauged by the melting point, if this is a hot molten material. For example, molten iron (m.p. = 1528°C) produces more intense burns than those due to molten lead (m.p. = 327°C); much of the heat is transferred during the solidification of the material (latent heat of fusion) and the total area of destruction, and prognosis, is determined before treatment is applied. It is for this reason that protection against eye trauma, as required by legislation, is so important in foundries; even if the eye is protected by the blink reflex of the eyelid, severe burning of these often results in cicatricial deformity and consequent exposure of the eye, which becomes inflamed (*exposure keratitis*) and eventually infected (*hypopyon ulcer*).

3. *Chemical burns* act entirely differently from heat. The tissues may eventually undergo coagulative necrosis, but the chemical action is progressive and the rate at which damage occurs depends on the type of chemical and its concentration. Immediate and efficient removal by irrigation and débridement can totally prevent permanent damage to the eye and vision.

a. *Coagulative and caustic substances* are mostly acid and alkalis.

Alkalis dissolve the fatty components of the epithelium and therefore penetrate more deeply than acids. The most destructive alkali commonly encountered is lime (quicklime or slaked lime); this penetrates both cornea and conjunctiva and then is deposited as insoluble calcium salts, which cannot be removed. Its immediate irrigation is therefore especially important, even if the specific chelating agent (sodium versonate) is unavailable.

b. *Detergents* are fat-dissolving substances (including alkalis). The non-alkalis such as soaps used to produce a painful but transient burn, but many of the modern synthetic detergents with additives are capable of not only penetrating the tissues but also producing permanent scarring and corneal opacity (leucoma).

c. *Antimetabolic substances* destroy by interfering with the intracellular chemistry, so that not only are cells destroyed, but other cells, though surviving, cannot undergo the replication required for healing. One of the first of these agents to be developed was the vesicant mustard gas and many of those patients exposed during the First World War were attending the ophthalmic outpatients until quite recently with a characteristic recurrent *keratitis*. Other mustards and antimetabolic agents are in the current reserves of war gases, but are also used in clinical medicine for the treatment of blood disorders such as *Hodgkin's disease*.

THE ASSESSMENT OF EYE INJURIES

Except in the case of severe injury with acute urgency for treatment, a history of the onset and progress of the condition should precede the examination of the eye. Eye injuries are often deceptively obvious ('black eye' or haemorrhage in the anterior chamber) so that a more serious aspect of injury (microscopic perforation and intra-ocular foreign body) is missed. A balanced assessment based on the history and the objective examination will usually prevent such omissions and the findings should be recorded on a casualty card such as that in Fig. 4.7.

History

In the assessment of trauma the history must be brief and to the point, directed to the causes as well as the consequences, which the patient will tend to emphasise. The history will usually be recent, but it is still important to itemise the events in order of occurrence, recording date and estimated times; only too often a patient will have delayed seeking advice and treatment with detriment to the prognosis. Pertinent questions help to elucidate the problem:

CASUALTY   CASUALTY No. **B**   **6791**   No. **B**   **6791**

FAMILY NAME	FORENAMES	UNIT No.
		DATE
		TIME
HOME ADDRESS		TELEPHONE No.
		M/S/W
OCCUPATION AND EMPLOYER	G.P.	AGE
		D.O.B.
PREVIOUS TREATMENT		ALLERGIES
WHERE TREATED		
V.A. WITH GLASSES c̄		V.A. WITHOUT GLASSES s̄
RIGHT LEFT	RIGHT LEFT	
HISTORY		NURSE'S REPORT

DATE _____

NAME _____

APPOINTMENT

DATE _____

TIME _____

AT * WOLVERHAMPTON EYE
       INFIRMARY
       COMPTON ROAD

   * CASUALTY UNIT
       TETTENHALL ROAD

   * DELETE AS NECESSARY

EXAMINATION
       RIGHT EYE   LEFT EYE

                    LIDS

            CONJUNCTIVA

                CORNEA

                    IRIS

                PUPIL

TREATMENT   BRING THIS SLIP

SISTERS SIGNATURE   FOLLOW UP
E.119

Fig. 4.7 Casualty record card (W.AHA)

1. Why did he first seek treatment? Was it because of the accident itself, the onset of pain, or visual defect?
2. Where did he first receive treatment? Was it at the works, industrial surgery, elsewhere, or is he only seeking it now?
3. When did the accident first happen?
4. How did the accident happen? What caused the accident? How did it develop?
   (The use of hammer and chisel or high-speed grinding should make the nurse suspect an intraocular foreign body; the exposure to chemicals, e.g. lime, indicates the need for urgent irrigation; the contamination by soil or injury by gardening tools may indicate likelihood of infection, especially *tetanus*.)
5. Was the patient using goggles or was other protection in use? Was the condition of the machine or tools good or poor?

6. Does the patient have a previous history of similar injury? Is this type of injury frequent in his occupation or in his place of work?

Avoid suggesting blame in your questioning; the precise cause of an injury usually lies in the interaction of many factors in which the employer's and the employee's responsibilities and the occupational hazards all play a part.

Subjective Examination

The examination of visual function is always by visual acuity, as described above, unless the patient is an infant or otherwise illiterate. With gross swelling of the eyelids it is normally possible gently to separate them sufficiently for the patient to read at least part of the test-type chart. Even in the most difficult cases, it should be possible to record a minimal visual response, even if it is only 'hand-movement' or 'perceives light'. The contraction of the pupil to light may indicate the retention of visual function.

Objective examination

The nurse is not usually expert in using the ophthalmoscope and the slit-lamp microscope, but these are so important in the ophthalmic examination that the opportunity to learn the simpler aspects of their use should not be missed. The nurse's examination will mostly be by naked eye or simple low-power magnification under sources of both diffuse and focal illumination. The examination starts with a general external assessment of the patient, both physical and mental; his general condition of awareness and consciousness may be indicative of head injury, or of drug intoxication. There may also be associated injuries to the face, head, or rest of his body. The ophthalmic examination itself starts with the superficial structures in sequence:

1. *Face and Eyelids.* The eyelids are protective and any injury which prevents closure is particularly dangerous; exposure and dessication of the cornea may lead to a perforating corneal ulcer. Swelling and oedema of the eyelids may be due to inflammation, allergy, and bruising, but in some cases the swelling may originate in the orbit (as with *orbital cellulitis*), in which case there is usually *proptosis* also. Small lacerations of the eyelid may sometimes be deeper than apparent at first examination and injuries of the upper eyelid by a spiked object have occasionally penetrated the roof of the orbit and brain. Dog bites often lead to an extensive loss of lid margin and in most countries the possibility of rabies must be remembered. Molten metal burns can lead to extreme loss of eyelid tissue with dangerous exposure of the eye.

Infection and inflammation of the lacrimal gland will produce swelling of the outer aspects of the upper eyelid; infection of the lacrimal sac produces swelling below the medial canthus and there may be a regurgitation of pus through the canaliculi when the swelling is gently pressed.

2. *Conjunctiva.* The structures behind the eyelids must be examined with great care. Not only can foreign matter and injury be hidden in the depths of the conjunctival fornices, but if there should be a perforation of the eye itself, pressure on the eye during examination could lead to a dangerous prolapse of the contents of the eye. The normal protective reflex of the facial muscles is to close the eyelids during examination and a quiet confidence is needed to enable the patient to relax as well as a proper technique by the nurse. In opening the eyelids the pressure should, as much as possible, be kept away from the eyes and onto the orbital margins, except where there is injury to the bone (Fig. 4.8).

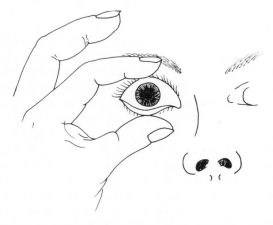

Fig. 4.8 Method of opening eyelids to inspect eye (thumb and forefinger outside orbital margin)

a. *The lower conjunctiva* is more readily exposed as the fornix is shallower and the lax skin can easily be drawn down by a finger on the centre of the lid below the eyelashes with gentle pressure towards the malar bone.

b. *The upper conjunctiva* can be difficult to examine as the fornix is deep. The bulbar conjunctiva is exposed by a finger above the eyelashes drawing the lid towards the supraorbital margin. Examination of the tarsal conjunctiva and fornix requires eversion of the lid.

c. Eversion of the upper eyelid is carried out in two ways, and in both the patient looks downward in order to relax the levator muscle. In one method the eyelid is seized with the thumb just below and the index finger above the margin and lashes (Fig. 4.9). The thumb draws the margin forwards away from the eye and rotates it over the tip of the index finger so that the top of the tarsal plate drops down behind the lid margin exposing the tarsal plate (Fig. 4.9 b and c).

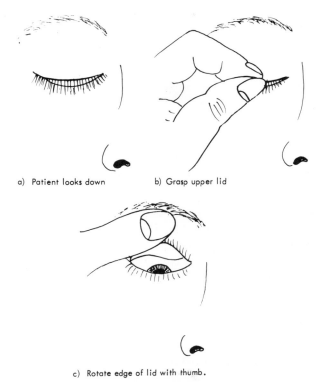

a) Patient looks down   b) Grasp upper lid

c) Rotate edge of lid with thumb.

Fig. 4.9 Eversion of eyelid to inspect upper fornix

The other method uses a glass rod or disposable applicator to assist the rotation by the index finger; the top of the rod is used to press the top of the tarsal plate downward. Double eversion for complete examination of the upper fornix requires the use of an eyelid retractor instead of a glass rod (Fig. 4.10).

The conjunctiva may be red due to contusion or haemorrhage, but redness often occurs with inflammation (*conjunctivitis, keratitis,*

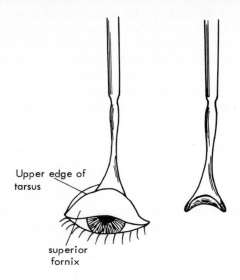

Upper edge of
tarsus

superior
fornix

Fig. 4.10 Eversion of eyelid over retractor

iritis), allergy, or in acute angle-closure *glaucoma*. Conjunctival laceration may sometimes involve the underlying globe. Foreign bodies often lodge under the upper eyelid or in the fornix.

3. *Cornea*. Corneal abrasions and ulcers are often extremely painful and may be associated with *photophobia* and *blepharospasm*. The nurse requires to become used to examining the cornea by focal illumination, which helps to differentiate the transparent cornea from the underlying pupil and iris. Corneal foreign bodies are common in the engineering industry, but corneal abrasions and small ulcers may be impossible to see without vital staining:

a. Fluorescin strips are applied to the lower conjunctival fornix, the dye dissolves in the lacrimal secretion, and it then stains abrasions of the cornea, as well as other defects in the epithelium, such as ulcers. The stain appears green and this is intensified if the illuminating light is passed through a cobalt-blue filter.

b. Rose-bengal eyedrops are used to stain diseased corneal epithelium including those cells in the margin of an ulcer. A punctate staining of the cornea may occur in virus-keratitis or with the dry cornea resulting from exposure or from atrophy of the lacrimal gland (*kerato-conjunctivitis sicca*). The contrast of the staining is intensified if the illuminating light is passed through a red-free filter.

The sensitivity of the cornea may be examined by a small wisp of cotton wool. The corneal sensation is impaired in diseases of the fifth cranial nerve (ophthalmic branch), including infections by *herpes simplex* (dendritic ulcer) and *herpes zoster*. The sensation is also impaired in deep coma.

4. *Pupil.* Pupils may be abnormal in size or shape. Unequal pupils usually occur as a result of treatment with mydriatic or miotic eyedrops, but an enlarged pupil associated with blood in the anterior chamber (*hyphaema*) results from a contusion injury.

An irregular pupil usually indicates adhesions to the lens (posterior synechiae) secondary to iritis. An iritis with pus in the anterior chamber (*hypopyon*) is usually due to infection and can result from a corneal ulcer with pyogenic microbes or a neglected perforating injury with or without an intraocular foreign body.

An oval semi-dilated pupil is characteristic of acute angle-closure *glaucoma*, when, during the acute attack, the eye is rock-hard, the conjunctiva flushed, and the cornea hazy.

5. *Lens.* Perforating injury to the eye with damage of the lens capsule will cause a cataract to develop with obvious impairment of vision.

Examination of the eye beyond the pupil requires an ophthalmoscope or other equipment, such as the slit-lamp, which will usually be the responsibility of the ophthalmologist. The ophthalmic nurse's examination of the eye should be limited to those details which are within her training and experience and especially those required for the routine casualty treatments, such as the removal of corneal foreign bodies, commonly delegated to the qualified ophthalmic nurse.

7. *Ocular movements.* Unless the vision of one eye has become impaired by injury, a recent onset of squint almost always will produce double vision (diplopia) for at least some directions of gaze. If only one muscle is weakened, the diplopia will usually be most evident when the patient looks in the direction produced by the normal contraction of that muscle (e.g. a leftward gaze for the left lateral rectus or the right medial rectus muscles). These squints almost always result from injury to the orbit or base of the brain and need further investigation, especially orthoptic and neurological.

THE TREATMENT OF EYE INJURIES

Many eye injuries require admission and treatment in the operating theatre. Casualty treatments described in this chapter are used for the less serious injuries or as urgent first aid preparatory to admission;

some are carried out by the nurse alone and others by the ophthalmologist assisted by a nurse.

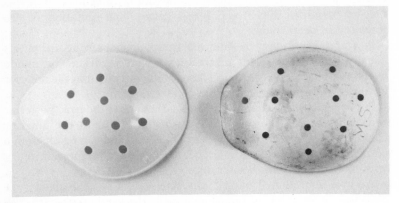

Fig. 4.11 Eye guards – cartella and Gluck's shield

1. *Principles of ophthalmic nursing treatments.* The eye is extraordinarily sensitive to light and to pressure and all treatments must be as gentle as is consistent with effectiveness. Pressure dressings must not be applied without an ophthalmologist's consent and in most cases it is more important to protect from pressure by the use of an eye guard or cartella (Fig. 4.11). Infection is catastrophic within the eye and all ophthalmic procedures should use a suitable clean technique:

a. *Antisepsis.* The nurse's hands must be washed thoroughly before and after every treatment using soap, brush and antiseptic washes.

b. *Asepsis.* All instruments and dressings must be fully sterilised before use. Packs from central sterilisation departments must be checked through for leaks and dates of sterilisation and not opened until required.

c. *Cross-infection.* Extra care is required if an infected case has just been treated or if the patient's other eye is infected. Infection can be air-borne with dust and treatments must not be carried out in a draughty room or within half an hour of domestic cleaning. Any domestic vacuum cleaner requires regular checking for the integrity of its dust filters together with bacteriological tests of the 'clean' side of the filter. Bacterial tests should also routinely include settle counts (from atmospheric particles) and control of sterilisers.

d. *Eyepads.* These have had an important place in the treatment of eye injuries and still have a limited application. A cartella eye shield applied with good quality adhesive tape gives better protection to the eye and the nurse is reminded that eyepads have distinct disadvantages:

(i) Abrasions can be produced if the patient opens his eyelids exposing the cornea to the back of the pad.

(ii) Infection can be promoted by the eyepad retaining any discharge and its warming effect on the surface of the ocular tissues.

(iii) Discomfort is produced if the eyepad is insecure and applied with insufficient pressure to prevent the blinking movement of the eyelashes.

(iv) Entropion may be increased in a susceptible subject.

(v) Burns are occasionally produced if the eyepad is ignited (usually by the patient).

Eyepads are mainly used after surgical procedures and are useful for immobilising the eyelid if sterile paraffin-gauze (tulle-gras) is applied directly to the lids beneath the pad. Eye bandages can be uncomfortable and have been almost totally replaced by the improved quality of adhesive tape (e.g. Blenderm). In an emergency a firm pad and bandage will always control bleeding from the orbit or eyelids, but must not be so firm as to endanger the blood supply to the optic nerve.

2. *First aid treatment carried out in casualty*

a. *Mechanical injuries.* Contusion injuries limited to the eyelids (black eye) may require no treatment beyond reassurance, but contusion of the eye itself or the orbit requires hospital admission.

Superficial abrasion of the conjunctiva or corneal epithelium requires the regular application of an antibiotic ointment (e.g. Oculentum chloramphenicol) during the healing process. If infection of the abrasion has occurred the patient will usually be admitted for treatment.

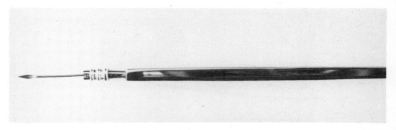

Fig. 4.12 Foreign body needle – Cluckie's (Dixey)

Small foreign bodies on the cornea or conjunctiva are usually superficial and may be lifted off the anaesthetised epithelium by the trained ophthalmic nurse using a small cotton wool swab. The deeper foreign body can usually be removed with a corneal needle (Fig. 4.12). The other requisites include an anaesthetic (e.g. Guttae amethocaine 0·5 per cent) and a speculum. The eyedrop is applied above the limbus so that it moistens the whole cornea. A speculum may be used to part the eyelids and expose the cornea. The corneal needle is potentially dangerous and shall only be used by those with practical training in its use; it is applied almost tangentially to the cornea to prevent the possibility of perforating the eye and the tip of the needle is brought into the corneal substance just deep to the foreign body. The nurse's hand is always steadied on the side of the patient's head; if the patient moves, the instrument in the nurse's hand will then move with the patient. After removal, antibiotic ointment is applied and the patient referred for examination within 24 hours. If the foreign body is iron, rust staining of the cornea will occur and the consequent 'rust-ring' may need removal later.

All deeper foreign bodies and serious lacerations of the ocular tissues require treatment by an ophthalmologist. Small lacerations may sometimes be sutured in casualty using the following equipment (Fig. 4.13):

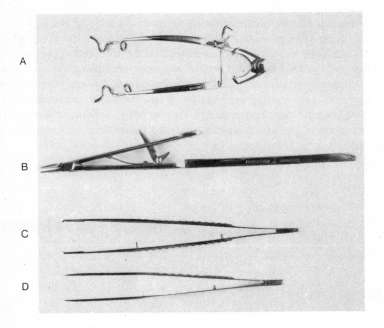

Fig. 4.13 Suturing instruments
  a. Clark's speculum
  b. Silcock needle holder
  c. Lister's forceps
  d. suture forceps (Moorfields)

Eye-speculum, suture 5/0 or 6/0 black silk (atraumatic needle), Silcock's needle holder, Lister's blocked-forceps, conjunctival forceps. sharp-pointed iris-scissors, drops, ointment, and dressings.

b. *Burns.* Thermal burns require little first aid, as either they are limited to a superficial reddening of the eyelids with no epithelial breaks and requiring no treatment, or the necrosis is so severe that admission is needed for surgical repair. The damage is fairly complete within the time of the injury.

In contrast, chemical burns require early (and repeated) first aid treatment as the damage produced by a chemical continues to intensify as long as the chemical is present. Irrigation by water will remove most chemicals, but in the casualty department isotonic saline (0·9 per cent) is used. A setting for irrigation (Fig. 4.14) will include:

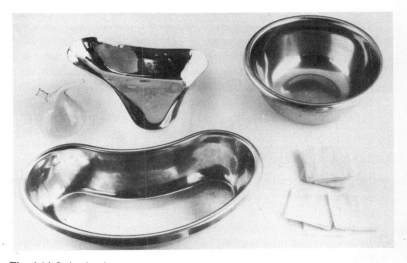

Fig. 4.14 Irrigating instruments
  a. undine
  b. Fisher's dish
  c. bowl and swabs
  d. receiver

Undine and stand for the lotion, Fisher's irrigation tray, a stainless steel measuring jug, bowl with eye swabs, receiver (or disposable paper bag) for used swabs. A cape is also required to protect the patient from splashes. Anesthetic eyedrops.

The lotion should not be warmed but used directly from a sealed container (as used for intravenous infusions). Whether sitting in a chair with headrest or lying on a couch, the patient's head needs to be nearly horizontal but inclined to the side to be irrigated. The nurse usually stands behind the patient and holds the eyelids apart with the fingers of one hand and pours out from the undine with the other hand. The irrigation dish receives the overflow and is held firmly against the cheek by either the patient himself or by an assistant. The flow of lotion is usually started on the cheek or side of the nose to accustom the patient to it before it flows directly on to the conjunctival sac. All aspects of the sac must be irrigated, double eversion of the upper eyelid being used when necessary. The flow must be steady and continuous, the patient being instructed to look to each side and up and down in order to expose the conjunctiva. After irrigation the eyelids are dried with a swab. Any particulate matter should be removed by irrigation assisted by a swab on a stick as needed.

Lime burns form insoluble particles both superficially and deep to the conjunctiva. These must be removed if possible and the deeper lime particles may be reduced by irrigation with a chelating lotion (sodium versonate 2·7 per cent). Early dilution of the lime is so important that tap water should be used rather than delay treatment. Later treatment of chemical burns may also include subconjunctival injection of saline to dilute the absorbed chemical.

OCCUPATIONAL HEALTH AND INDUSTRIAL OPHTHALMOLOGY

Many patients attending the eye casualty for treatment will have been referred directly from work with occupational trauma. The casualty nurses therefore see the results of occupational hazards and the casualty should be concerned to maintain a close liaison with industry and a feedback of information, so that protection from these hazards will be improved.

Occupational health is particularly important in modern industry, which demands high standards of quality and productivity in order to maintain high wages not possible in the less developed economies. Vision contributes to the control of many modern machines and it is important that the standards of vision are assessed before such work is undertaken; as well as the visual acuity required to read instructions and gauges and for measurement, a full field of vision is needed. In many industries such as textiles, colour vision is required as well as in those industries using colour signals and codes, e.g. railways, air-traffic control, and electronics. Chronic eye diseases such as allergic *blepharoconjunctivitis* and chronic infections (*trachoma*,

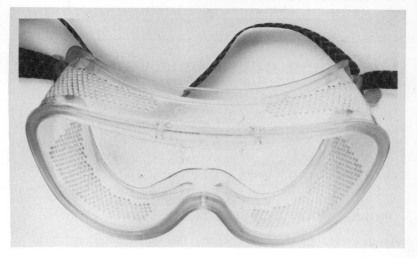

Fig. 4.15 Protective goggles

haemophilus *conjunctivitis*) may result in undue sensitivity to fumes and dust; also the factory atmosphere, if hot, dusty and poorly ventilated, may contribute to the persistence of these infections.

Industrial ophthalmology is often carried out by the industrial nurse under the responsibility of a works doctor. In many industries eye injury and disability is so important that these nurses should maintain a close liaison with the casualty of the ophthalmic hospital or unit and, as necessary, attend clinical tuition and gain wider experience of these injuries. There are many hazards to the eye in industry and wherever necessary these can be reduced by the wearing of protective goggles (Fig. 4.15) or protection built into the machines themselves. Some of the more important hazards include:

1. Water or any form of damp in a foundry; if there is any spillage of molten metal the water will evaporate explosively.
2. Fast revolving machines, such as capstans, lathes and grinders, develop large centrifugal forces which can throw particles towards the eye at very high velocities.
3. Chemical fumes, such as occur with rayon-spinning, cause irritation of the eyes unless efficient exhaust ventilation is provided.
4. Hammer and chisel work quite often results in an intraocular foreign body when a small fragment of metal flies off the brittle hammer or chisel.
5. Interior decorating especially when plastering the ceiling, can be the cause of lime burns. Apart from building, lime is used in agriculture and may affect the quarry workers where it is obtained.

Outpatient ophthalmic nursing

ORGANISATION AND FUNCTION

As described in the last chapter, the outpatient department is alternative to the casualty department as a portal of entry for patients obtaining access to hospital services. Patients attending as outpatients will usually have planned appointments whether referred directly from the casualty, from general practitioners, or from other hospital clinics. The prime purpose of the department is to provide a second opinion on the patients' eye diseases, but this also entails a need for many specialised investigations and treatments. The fact that many patients continue to attend an outpatients department for a follow-up surveillance for many years is mainly due to the technical complexity and expense of ophthalmic equipment, which cannot be available to the general practitioner.

Ophthalmic outpatients departments have a rather singular relationship to general practitioners, who are responsible for the primary care in most other areas of medicine. Such is the specialisation of ophthalmic knowledge and techniques that most eye conditions are not only referred at an early stage to a hospital clinic for diagnosis but also the surveillance and treatment is continued there until the condition is resolved. The ophthalmic clinic is therefore responsible for the whole care of eye diseases and the outpatient department undertakes the role of providing for diagnosis and treatment. Some patients attend over a period of many years and are investigated in the special diagnostic clinics or admitted for investigation, treatment and surgery as required; with the records department the outpatient clinic represents the organisation required for this continuous surveillance of the patients' disabilities and it is therefore important that the nurse should better understand its role and participate in its work.

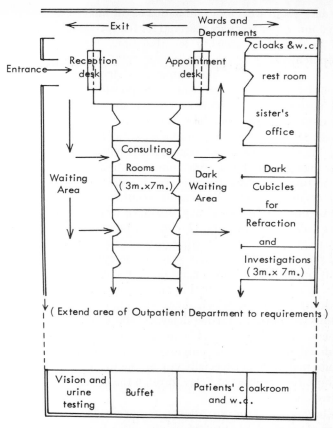

Fig. 5.1 Ophthalmic outpatient department (outline scheme with patient flow)

The structure of a typical ophthalmic outpatients may be illustrated by Fig. 5.1. The reception area includes the waiting area with the appointments and records counter, the transport office, and medical social worker; this area is mainly under the control of the senior records officer and it is important that the nurses and records staff work in co-operation so that the patients can pass between this area and the clinical area without difficulty or undue delay.

The clinical area of the outpatients department has traditionally been of an open plan; most modern clinics are divided to provide more privacy although this may make the teaching and supervision of trainee specialists more difficult, and it also can make supervision by the nurses more difficult. Note that the clinic includes well-illuminated areas for the initial examination and history-taking and dark-room areas for examination of the interior of the eye and for refraction; other areas are reserved for the special clinics, where there will be sufficient security for the more expensive and delicate equipment.

The *organisation* of the outpatients department is maintained largely by the nursing staff, who are responsible for its equipment and will ensure that the patients receive the attention they require. Although patients attending ophthalmic outpatients departments usually receive a single appointment date and time, this may involve a large number of tests and examinations within the clinic before and after being seen by a consultant ophthalmologist or one of his supporting staff. New patients are especially likely to be delayed; all patients usually have a visual acuity recorded before being seen by the doctor but new patients may also have urine, blood pressure, and intraocular pressure tests. Having examined the patient, the doctor may request a variety of further tests such as visual fields, orthoptic, and refraction. All this may involve the patient joining the end of many queues and it is important that the supervising staff ensure that there is no undue delay within any one of these queues. The use of mydriatic eyedrops which dilate the pupil to examine the ocular fundus will impose a further delay and this should be explained to the patient, who should be able to relax in a comfortable area while mydriasis develops. The complex queue structure of most ophthalmic clinics makes them especially vulnerable to any staff absence, which will produce protracted delay through the clinic unless detected and corrected.

The *function* of the outpatients, as described above, is central to the work of the whole eye unit providing both a diagnostic service and also continuous care for patients with eye disease. It is within the outpatients department that the clinical ophthalmologist will most often make not only a diagnosis but also other decisions regarding investigation, treatment and surgery, which will affect the future care of the patient, whether admitted to the ward or not. It is therefore important that the ophthalmic nurse is conversant with the decision-making processes in the outpatient department.

Communication to the nurse, as to the patient, is most commonly by mouth and any ambiguity or misunderstanding should be eliminated by enquiry. However, it is vital that all important decisions are recorded (as described in Chapter 3) on the patient's record case-sheet, since these bring together in a permanent document the clinical details, the diagnosis and future planning for investigation and treatment; the nurse should use these records to check on the patient's requirements. As the patient passes to each clinical area within the outpatients department, his record forms the basic communication system used by all those responsible for his clinical care.

THE ROLE OF THE NURSE IN OUTPATIENTS

Outwardly it might seem that the nurse working in the outpatients department does work which could as well be done by a clerk or administrator. However, the needs of the patient make it essential that the control of the department is within the responsibility of someone with detailed clinical experience. In Britain the senior nurse has accepted this role although in many countries with less developed nursing services the doctor himself still maintains the continuous management responsibility for his clinic. The role of the ophthalmic nurse will require:

1. Management skills, including ability to delegate and assign work, to control queues and groups, planning, budget-control, and reporting.
2. Clinical knowledge which is wide enough to understand the decision-making processes of the department and to respond to the patients' queries.
3. Nursing skills required to provide outpatient treatment and the equipment for minor outpatient surgery.
4. Simple technical knowledge, especially in optics and electricity, in order to understand the purpose and use of ophthalmic equipment and its maintenance.
5. Aspects of community ophthalmology and sociology sufficient to understand the interaction of the outpatients department not only with the rest of the hospital but also with general practice and other areas of community and occupational care.

THE GENERAL OPHTHALMIC CLINIC

The outpatient clinic is equipped for the basic diagnostic procedures and the nurse should understand the use and care of the equipment in relation to the diagnostic process. The principles in the care of equipment are detailed in Chapter 9, but it should be remembered that most ophthalmic equipment is a combination of optical elements (for viewing) and electrical (for illumination). Mains voltage is dangerous and most instruments either use a transformer reducing the voltage to 6 or 12 volts, or use two torch batteries in series giving a voltage of 3 volts. It is important to experience the use of this equipment to learn its properties and also to use the supplier's catalogues to examine alternative equipment available. Basically very little equipment is needed:

1. *Subjective examination* requires a visual-acuity chart, a case of trial lenses with trial frame, small targets (or fingers) for confrontation field test, Maddox rod and wing for testing ocular imbalance, and colour vision charts.

2. *Objective examination* requires a good general illumination for the initial examination, a slit-lamp microscope for detailed examination, an ophthalmoscope for examination of the internal eye, and a retinoscope for examination of the refractive power of the eye. A small light-source for transillumination is also required (for diagnosis of tumours).

The details given below will usually only be meaningful if the equipment being described is to hand.

The equipment is manufactured in a variety of designs and it is important to learn from a catalogue those alternatives available and compare the advantages and disadvantages of the equipment with that used in your own clinic.

Subjective examination

1. *Visual acuity charts*

These have been referred to in the chapter on casualty work, and include Snellen's non-serif type for distance, the Faculty of Ophthalmologists reading type for near, and a variety of illiteracy charts. The visual acuity without and with glasses must be recorded at every visit.

2. *Trial lenses*

These are available in a case containing spherical lenses (plus for convex, minus for concave) ranging from 0·12 to at least 20 dioptres and plus and minus cylindrical lenses ranging from 0·25 to 6 dioptres. The case contains prisms for measuring the angle of ocular balance between the two eyes and also the following:

a. A pin-hole for improvement of visual acuity without spectacles. In the absence of spectacles a pin-hole (c̄P.H) visual acuity should be recorded.

b. A stenopoeic slit for improvement of vision in cases of *astigmatism*; the slit is rotated to produce the best acuity.

c. A Maddox rod to be used with a spot light; through the rod the spot appears as a thin red line separated from the spot in proportion to the degree of ocular imbalance (or latent *squint*). The strength of prism required to bring the line on to the spot is a measure of the imbalance.

d. Two colour filters, red and green, used to dissociate the eyes in other tests of ocular balance.

These lenses now conform to a British Standard (BS 3010). Most modern trial lenses are of a reduced aperture; the wider rim allows handling without touching of the glass, which must always be kept clean and polished.

3. Trial frame

The trial frame is designed to take a combination of trial lenses in front of each eye, usually up to four, and it should be comfortable, light and sturdy. These requirements are to an extent in conflict and the more robust frames are not so much used now as they are found to be too heavy. The frames are easily distorted and should be checked for this.

4. Small targets

The small targets used in the general examination are usually 'hat-pins' with coloured rounded heads (white, red, green). These can be available in a small 'pin-cushion' and used for assessment of the patient's visual field; the patient looks straight ahead at the examiner's nose or eye, and the head of the pin is slowly brought inwards from the extreme side until the patient notices it (without moving his eyes). This is repeated from each side and above and below until the examiner is satisfied as to the extent of any loss of visual field present. The Amsler chart is used for assessing changes in the central field.

5. Maddox wing and Maddox rod

The Maddox rod has been described. The wing uses a vertical bar of metal to separate the visual objects seen by each eye; the right eye sees the arrows and the left the numbers. With no common target for sight the eyes can relax into a position relative to one another determined by the degree of ocular imbalance. This is shown by the movement of the arrows in relation to the numbers and the numbers to which the arrows eventually point give a measure of the degree of imbalance between the eyes (white for horizontal imbalance and red for vertical).

6. Colour vision test

There are a large number of methods for testing colour vision and the most generally useful in the clinic is the Ishihara chart; this consists of numbers made up of coloured dots. The ability to read the numbers depends on the normality of colour vision; this test is fairly sensitive for diagnosing between red and green blindness, but not for blue blindness, which is very rare.

Objective examination

1. General illumination

This needs to be adequate but, since it also requires to be flexible and controlled by a thyristor-dimmer, an incandescent source is to be preferred to fluorescent. A diffuse 'flat' illumination is adequate during the preliminary history-taking and examination of the general appearance of the patient, his face and surface ocular structures.

The cornea acts as a convex mirror and may produce confusing images unless the sources of illumination are placed well above the patient's head and dimmed when required.

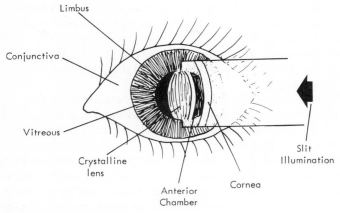

Fig. 5.2 Slit lamp view of eye

2. *Slit-lamp examination*

Although the slit-lamp microscope was devised by Gullstrand to produce the narrow-beam examination of an optical section of the eye (Fig. 5.2), it has now become the ophthalmologist's general-purpose microscope for the examination of the eye and its anterior adnexa back to the retina and optic disc. The use of contact lenses, which reduce the focal power of the cornea, enables the ophthalmologist to examine the angle of the eye (gonioscope, Fig. 5.10), and the central and peripheral retina (three-mirror contact lens). Although mechanically one system, the slit-lamp microscope is best understood as two co-ordinated parts (Fig. 5.3):

a. a binocular microscope producing a magnification of about × 10 to × 20.

b. an illuminating source with a condensing focal system controlled by a variable slit as well as a rotating disc with a choice of diaphragm sizes or coloured filters.

These two parts move together as a mechanical unit and can be rotated in relation to each other round a central pillar. The pillar and other moving parts require regular attention (cleaning and a little oiling) if they are to move easily. The surfaces of all lenses and mirrors must

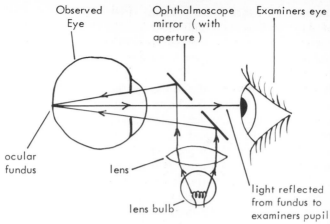

Fig. 5.3 Optics of ophthalmoscope

also be kept clean but *never* oiled: the lamp-bulb may be replaced when it burns out or loses efficiency by 'sooting' inside the glass of the bulb. If the lamp is left on or regularly over-loaded (7·5 volts for a 6 volt bulb), its life is considerably shortened by the consequent overheating. The safety of the equipment is greatly increased by the transformer, which reduces the voltage for the mains (230 volts in the U.K.) to about 6 volts, but the construction is mostly metallic and should always be earthed. Dust and dirt reduce the efficiency of the focusing system, and also of the electric switches, so that the equipment must always be covered and switched off at the wall when not in use.

3. *Ophthalmoscope*

The interior of the eye behind the lens was invisible to clinicians until the invention of the ophthalmoscope by Babbage and von Helmholtz in the middle of the nineteenth century. This enlarged view of the eye and its diseases was a most important factor in the development of modern ophthalmology and the ophthalmic nurse is advised to obtain at least some acquaintance with the use of an ophthalmoscope in order to understand its contribution to the examination of an eye. As with the slit-lamp, the ophthalmoscope has two parts – a viewing system with lenses and an illuminating system using a lamp-bulb which may be powered by a dry battery (usually 3 volts) or by the mains through a transformer; the handle of a mains ophthalmoscope can become hot and a recent development is a *fibre-optic* ophthalmoscope, in which the light source is connected to the ophthalmoscope by a flexible fibre-optic cable. To view the fundus of the eye it is essential that the observer examine the eye in a direction coincident with the light-beam (Fig. 5.3), which is why the observer usually looks through a hole in the mirror. As with the slit-lamp, cleanliness of the whole instrument is important and it should be returned to its case when not in use.

4. *Retinoscope*

This has an appearance similar to the ophthalmoscope, but it is constructed to produce a long-focus beam, being used at half to one metre from the patient's eyes. The light reflected from the fundus of the eye is examined at this distance and its movement neutralised by lenses, which can then indicate the refractive power of the eye and estimate the spectacle lenses required for correction of a refractive error. It must also be kept clean and the dry-batteries renewed as necessary.

5. *Transillumator*

This equipment is very often needed to allow light to be focused near the back of the eye, through which the light passes. This test does help to distinguish, for example, a simple retinal detachment from one due to a solid tumour. The light probe is usually a 'cold lite' or *fibre-optic* construction; both use the principle of total internal reflection.

SPECIAL CLINICS

The diagnosis of a specific disease often requires specialised skills and equipment, which in general medicine are often provided by the various pathological laboratories. Ophthalmologists also use these facilities as appropriate, but have developed specialised techniques which may be required in ophthalmology only; these include campimetry (visual field measurement) and fluorescin angiography, and clinics specialising in the diagnosis of glaucoma, squint, orbital disease, retinal detachment, corneal disease, diabetic disease, and others. These clinics are sometimes grouped together near the outpatients and controlled by the outpatient nursing staff, but in other hospitals they may be dispersed with an increased burden on organisation. Orthoptics and the treatment of squint is controlled by the orthoptists and not the nursing staff.

1. *Orthoptic department*

The orthoptic department is concerned with the diagnosis and treatment of squint and ocular imbalance; it is staffed by specialist orthoptists, who are responsible to the consultant staff. Although it is outside the outpatient nursing responsibility, the traffic of patients, especially children, between the two departments is considerable so that it is important that the nurse has some knowledge of orthoptics. There may also be areas of overlapping organisation and co-operation, such as the use of a common play waiting area for the children, and communication of test results back to the medical staff.

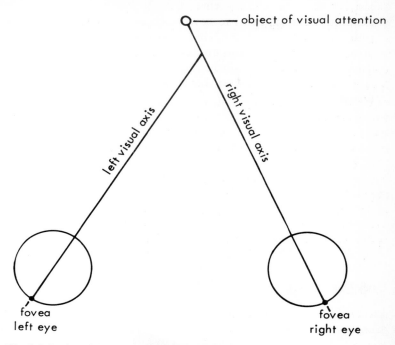

Fig. 5.4 Squint with deviation of left visual axis

A squint can be defined (Fig. 5.4) as a condition in which the two visual axes do not pass through the object of visual attention simultaneously. The definition includes:

a. Unilateral squint, in which the visual axis of the squinting eye is never directed at the object of attention.

b. Alternating squint, in which the visual axis used can switch between the right and left eye alternately.

The diagnosis of squint is based on history and symptoms, examination, and specialised investigation:

a. The subjective history is most often related by the parents, although in adults with recent onset of squint, *diplopia* (double vision) may be the main symptom. In children there is usually a suppression of the confusing double image and the squint is noted by either the parents, clinic doctor, or other acquaintances. There is often a family history of squint or refractive error.

b. The objective examination includes an examination of ocular movement, as may be obtained by the following of a torch-light, and various tests which dissociate the use of binocular vision. The simplest of these tests is the cover-test, in which the back of the examiner's hand is used to cover each eye alternately while the patient looks at a test object. This manoeuvre accentuates the movement of each eye as it takes up fixation and is the basic test used to detect squint and to estimate the size of the squint (Fig. 5.5). Although most squints are horizontal, vertical squints are not uncommon.

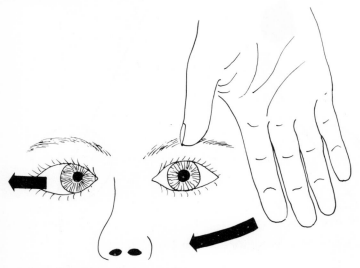

Right eye fixes object as hand covers left eye.

Fig. 5.5 Cover test examination

c. The further investigation of squint in the orthoptic department uses a variety of specialised instruments. These are used to measure the angle of squint or to estimate the quality of binocular vision:

(i) The *Hess or the Lee's screen* is used to estimate the angle of squint while the eyes are moved into the horizontal and vertical directions of gaze. It shows how the angle varies with the direction of gaze and may therefore be used to diagnose the paralysis of one or more ocular muscles, but both eyes need to be used without suppression of either ocular image.

(ii) the *synoptophore* presents an illuminated image to each eye separately and the image may be varied by the use of selected pairs of transparent slides. These slides (Fig. 5.6) have been selected to diagnose the presence of (a) simultaneous perception without sup-

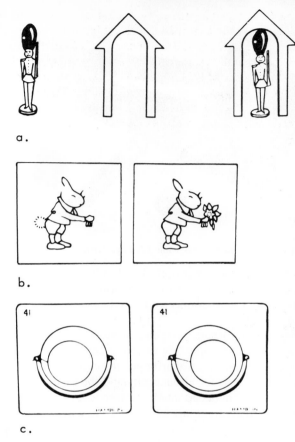

a.

b.

c.

Fig. 5.6 Synoptophore slides
  a. simultaneous macular perception
  b. fusion
  c. stereopsis

pression of either image (b) the quality of binocular fusion of the image, and (c) the presence of stereoscopic vision. The synoptophore allows the direction of the images to be varied in order to assess the range over which the eye will converge and diverge while maintaining binocular fusion, when this is present. Diplopia may indicate loss of fusion but if suppression occurs one eye will move off the axis for viewing the slide while the other eye maintains fixation of of the object of attention.

(iii) Other instruments used include prisms for bending the visual axis, the lenses of the trial frame, and the Maddox rod and Maddox wing (Fig. 5.7).

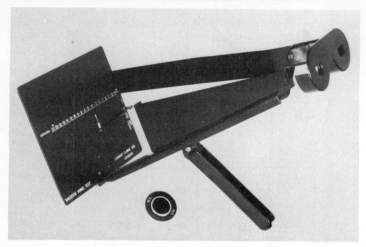

Fig. 5.7 Maddox rod and Maddox wing (Clement Clarke)

Most of this equipment is optical and only works efficiently when kept clean and free from dust. Electrical equipment needs special care and should be disconnected from the mains supply when being cleaned.

d. The prognosis of squint depends as much on visual function as on the angle of squint, especially in young children, who are liable to develop *amblyopia*. Much of orthoptic testing depends on the use of a wide variety of tests for visual acuity and the treatment of squint in young children is aimed as much at improving visual acuity as at correcting the angle of squint, which is usually marginal. With early detection and treatment the prognosis for squint can be good, although a squint dating from birth rarely achieves binocular fusion of the visual image; careful management of the condition, including occlusion of the fixing eye, should achieve a useful and often normal acuity for the squinting eye.

In adults the prognosis usually depends on the diplopia, which is relieved at first by the use of an occlusive patch. Binocular vision needs to be maintained and the use of prisms may achieve this by their alteration of the visual direction. If the squint has become constant, surgical correction will usually be needed, depending on the cause of the squint, which may be due to trauma, orbital disease, inflammatory, vascular, and neoplastic disease of the central nervous system, etc.

2. *Visual field (campimetry) clinic*

The examination of the visual field is a subjective exercise requiring considerable concentration by both the patient and the examiner; it cannot usually be performed with either accuracy or convenience in the main outpatients department unless this is the type which provides considerable quiet and privacy. The principles of campimetry depend on the normal range of retinal acuity, which is greatly reduced at the periphery. It follows that the size of the normal visual field can be increased by using a larger test object or by a brighter ambient illumination, up to a limit imposed by the total size of the retina and the optics of the eye. In many diseases, such as *glaucoma*, the adaptation to dark is defective and a moderate reduction of illumination will emphasise pathological changes in the visual field.

The dark room used for campimetry may contain a variety of instruments, but the control of illumination requires to be accurate through the use of a dimmer-switch for the ceiling lights and a dull non-reflective wall paint. The instruments may include:

a. *A perimeter*, which is intended to assess the whole field and therefore has an arc or bowl coming round to the side of the head at least to a 100 degree angle to the axis of visual fixation. The target size can be varied and white is used almost always; a choice of colours (red, blue, green) is often provided as colour-loss scotomas may occur in neurological disease and toxic amblyopia (e.g. tobacco). As the target moves in an arc, its radius to the eye is constant and its apparent size remains the same; its brightness depends on an even and controlled illumination, which can be accurately calibrated in the more expensive perimeters (Goldman, Gambs, etc.).

b. *A tangent screen*, which is most frequently the Bjerrum screen (Fig. 5.8). This is a plain black screen, 2 metres square, flat to a wall, and tangential to the arc of the visual field. The periphery of the screen is further from the eye and targets therefore tend to be visually smaller there. The size of the screen is limited to the testing of the central field within 30 degrees from the fixation point. The screen requires even illumination and the patient fixes a central white spot, while sitting 2 metres from it.

Many other visual field analyses have been devised such as the Fieldmaster (a computerised random selection of targets) and Friedmann (a varied pattern of targets) and various combinations of illumination, colour, size, contrast, etc. can make the field examination complex and time consuming. However, the diagnostic use of the test is to identify the characteristic field loss in various diseases and, as explained in Chapter 2, this is principally determined by the anatomy of the visual pathway. A simple approach to testing of fields is clinically often quite sufficient and does not overstretch the patient's co-operation. In some cases the direct confrontation test

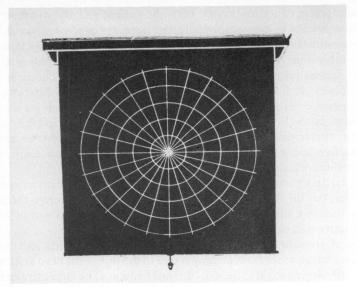

Fig. 5.8 Tangent (Bjerrum) screen

comparing the patient's field with one's own by means of a pin's head or even fingers can sometimes demonstrate the significant field-loss.

The nurse will need to know the conditions required for accurate visual field examination with special attention to the control of the illumination and the cleanliness of the equipment; a white target is no longer white if discoloured and under imperfect illumination. The patient requires a comfortable and stable seat and clean eyepads will be supplied to occlude the eye not under test.

3. *Fluorescin angiography*

Fluorescin angiography depends on the property of fluorescin in blue light to fluoresce green. A 5 per cent to 10 per cent solution of fluorescin is injected into a vein in the arm and the fluorescence photographed as it passes through the vessels of the retina and choroid (sometimes the iris or conjunctiva). This method gives a very much more detailed record of the vascular structure than is possible by ordinary retinal photography and is therefore used to help the diagnoses of conditions affecting the circulation, principally the *retinopathies*. In diabetic retinopathies minute aneurysms may be discovered long before they become apparent with the ophthalmoscope.

The camera used to record the passage of fluorescin through the eye has a motor-driven camera-back and the patient's head needs to be kept quite still while the successive exposures are made with high-intensity flash. The patient should be comfortable with the headrest carefully adjusted. The patient often feels weak and nauseated after the injection and should be sat in a low easy chair for recovery; he may be reassured that the yellow staining of the skin will disappear after a few hours. In some patients, particularly diabetics, the arm veins can be small and difficult to inject; if this is so they may be dilated by immersing the arm in hot water before the investigation.

The nurse will need to provide a set of instruments on a tray for the doctor performing the angiography. This will be for the injection of the dye and include sterile skin-cleaning swabs with antiseptic solution (separate or impregnated), arm constricting band (to dilate the veins) and materials for injection (syringe, ampoule of sterilised 5 per cent or 10 per cent fluorescin, intravenous needle, adhesive plaster disc). An adequate stock of film, both colour and high speed black-and-white must always be available. The nurse should explain the procedure to the patient, who will require to attend about an hour beforehand for the instillation of mydriatic eyedrops; he will need to know that his skin will go slightly yellow and the colour will be eliminated through the urine.

4. *Glaucoma investigation*

The diagnosis (or exclusion) of glaucoma requires a range of tests beyond the ordinary history and examination in the general eye clinic. Glaucoma simplex is the commonest type of *glaucoma* and is insidious in onset, being usually symptomless. The patient is often referred at the time of a routine spectacle test when the optician has noted a cupping of the optic disc or a restriction of visual field; loss of acuity occurs late and heralds an impending blindness. Acute forms of glaucoma with high intraocular pressure and pain are more obvious in their diagnosis. The investigation used in the special clinic includes:

a. Examination of the optic disc with an ophthalmoscope or slit-lamp to determine its shape and size and the proportion that is cupped.

b. Visual acuity and field examinations as described in campimetry (2. above). The characteristic field loss is an arcuate scotoma (Fig. 5.9) with a horizontal limit medial to the point of fixation.

c. Gonioscopy is an examination of the drainage angle of the anterior chamber using a contact lens containing a mirror (Fig. 5.10). In many types of glaucoma obstruction to the flow of aqueous in the angle causes the increased intraocular pressure but in glaucoma simplex the angle is open and the obstruction is in the tissues beyond the angle.

d. Tonometry estimates the intraocular pressure. Although an approximate estimate can be gained by digital palpation of an eye, the

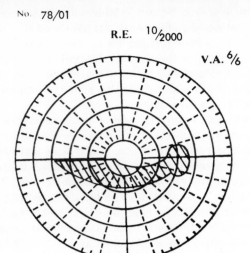

Fig. 5.9 Arcuate scotoma

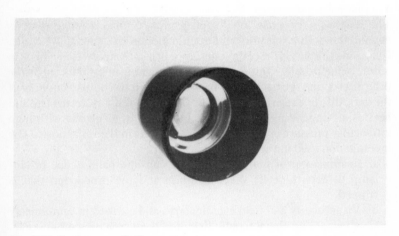

Fig. 5.10 Gonioscope – Goldman

small differences that can occur in glaucoma cannot. The normal intraocular pressure is 15 ± 5 mmHg and a clinical tonometer needs to be accurate to ± 1 mmHg differences. The commonly used Schiotz tonometer did not achieve this, as it was based on a measurement of indentation calibrated for pressure on cadaveric and animal eyes. The Goldmann's applanation tonometer, which flattens the centre of the cornea, measures the force required to produce a standard area of applanation (diameter = 3·06 mm) and the pressure measurement is directly obtained by calculation:

$$Pressure = Force \div Area$$

At the chosen area Pressure (mmHg) = Force (Gm-wt) multiplied by 10. The Goldmann tonometer needs to be used with the slit-lamp microscope, and a more portable tonometer (the Perkin's) is based on the same principle and can be used on recumbent patients. Tonometry involves contact with the human cornea and can therefore be a route of cross infection; cleaning of the tonometer head after use and its sterilisation with antiseptic solution is important.

e. Tonography estimates the change of intraocular pressure during prolonged use of a Schiotz tonometer. For greater accuracy and in order to produce a paper-trace (tonogram) an electronic Schiotz tonometer is used. The weight of the tonometer forces up the intra-ocular pressure, which returns to normal more quickly in a normal than in a glaucomatous eye. This rate of return to normal is considered to be related mainly to the condition of the aqueous outflow channels and is used to calculate the coefficient of facility of aqueous outflow, C (an abnormal C is less than $0·1$ mm^3 sec^1 mmHg^1 as explained in Chapter 2). The electronic tonometer is extremely sensitive (to within $0·005$ mm of the plunger movement) and regular servicing as well as scrupulous cleaning of the tonometer is essential.

f. Provocative tests are based on physiological conditions which elevate the intraocular pressure in glaucoma. In the water drinking test, the patient, who will have been starved of fluid and solids for four hours, drinks one litre of water (flavoured) and the intraocular pressure is estimated before and at regular intervals for two hours after. In glaucoma simplex the pressure often increases by 5 mmHg or more. The use of mydriatic drops, such as homatropine or cyclopentolate, produces a similar increase of pressure in angle-closure glaucoma, as the retracted iris blocks the narrow angle of the anterior chamber.

The variety of tests available for glaucoma has improved the diagnosis of doubtful cases, and it is important that the results are recorded in a permanent and accessible manner.

The nurse will need to know in broad outline the techniques employed in a glaucoma clinic and to give simple explanations to the patient as required, as for example when preparing the patient for the water drinking test or other provocative tests. The results of the tests should be explained to the patient by the doctor responsible for the continuing management of the treatment.

Sterilisation is important as much of the equipment such as the gonioscope and tonometer head comes into contact with the patient's cornea. The nurse will make sure that for each slit-lamp or tonometer in use there will be sufficient anaesthetic and lubricating eyedrops (e.g. benoxinate and hypromellose) and also antiseptic solution and medical tissues for wiping the area of contact of the gonioscopes and tonometers. It is essential to use an antiseptic which is not harmful to the acrylic material and a 0·1 per cent aqueous solution of phenyl hydrargyrum boricum (Merfen) is frequently used. Cleaning is also needed to maintain the optical surfaces smooth and transparent and all equipment should be checked for this before and after use in the clinic.

Many larger hospitals employ glaucoma technicians to perform tonometry, tonography and campimetry, but even here the nurse may continue to exercise an important role in the organisation of the clinic and co-ordination of patient care.

5. *Orbital disease*

Most orbital diseases produce *proptosis* but as the orbit is beyond the view of the ophthalmoscope and contains tissue not visible on ordinary x-ray examination, many special techniques have been used in the diagnosis of orbital disease. The careful recording of the proptosis on successive visits using an exophthalmometer can demonstrate a change not discernable by the naked eye. The normal straight x-ray examination will show up most diseases involving the bones, but other techniques (some radiological) are used to locate orbital disease more accurately:

a. Radiological techniques include:

Tomography, in which all x-ray shadows within a calculated plane are defined, is used to demonstrate small orbital fractures on the optic foramen.

Oxygen injection behind the eye is used to define soft-tissue outlines in this area.

Venography by injection of the orbital veins demonstrates their pattern, which can be distorted by tumours and vascular disease.

Computerised tomography (EMI-scan) is a recent development for measuring the absorption of x-rays by various tissues and can therefore distinguish abnormal soft-tissue lesions in the orbit.

b. Ultrasonography is a technique based on the reflected echoes of *high-frequency* (8–12 MHz) sound. Structures not visible by conventional x-ray methods reflect sound and can therefore be detected.

c. Orbitonometry is a method used to measure the elastic resilience of the tissues; this is increased in the more severe types of dysthyroid exophthalmos.

6. Other special clinics

There may often be specialised diagnostic clinics for the investigation of retinal detachment, uveitis, corneal disease, etc. As with the other clinics, all these areas of investigation require specialised equipment and techniques and the nurse should aim to become conversant with at least the aims of the various clinics, as well as the nature and care of the equipment.

a. In *retinal detachment* the success of surgery usually depends on an accurate assessment of the hole or tear in the retina and its location. Special charts for mapping the retinal detachment are therefore used, and the retina will be examined by both the direct and indirect ophthalmoscope and also, sometimes, the slit-lamp using a contact lens.

b. *Uveitis* is often due to systemic disease so that investigation will be aimed at elucidating any systemic aetiology through a general examination of the patient, and laboratory and x-ray examination. Evidence of general inflammatory disease should be looked for, and this may be confirmed by an increased ESR (erythrocyte sedimentation rate), increase in white cell count, or an increase in the level of antibodies to various pathogens such as Streptococcus and Toxoplasma. This clinic will involve the co-ordinated services of a general physician and the hospital laboratories together with the ophthalmologist.

c. *Corneal disease* may often have a fairly obvious diagnosis as with corneal abscess or dendritic ulcer. Other types of keratitis, often due to virus, and other corneal diseases may be more difficult to diagnose and require both detailed investigations and careful management. Investigations will include bacteriology and virology in *keratitis*, and the careful assessment of the effect of the corneal disease on vision. Corneal *astigmatism* can often be corrected by contact lenses if spectacles are not helpful.

Trachoma is an important cause of severe visual defect in the poorer nations and is due to infection with a virus-like agent, Chlamydia; the infection tends to be chronic with exacerbations, so that management will require not only treatment, but also continued surveillance and the tracing of contacts in the family. A corneal disease clinic may also assess the need for surgical treatment and various types of corneal graft. This type of special clinic provides the opportunity for concentrating many diagnostic and therapeutic skills on each clinic problem.

d. *A contact lens fitting* department can be an important adjunct to the work of the corneal clinic. The contact lens has developed over the last century from a crude blown-glass cup to the modern custom-fitted plastic lens, and in Britain today the majority are supplied for the correction of simple refractive errors and worn for cosmetic reasons. Nevertheless the contact lens has an important place in therapy and typical applications include:

(i) *High refractive errors* for which the conventional spectacle-lens produces too large a change in image size and also image distortion.

(ii) *High astigmatism* due to corneal disease including keratoconus and not correctable by spectacle lenses.

(iii) *Blepharoptosis* as a support to the upper eyelid.

(iv) *Exposure keratitis* as a protection to the cornea when the eyelids fail to cover, as after burns.

(v) *Unilateral aphakia*, as a single aphakic spectacle-lens produces too much magnification for binocular fusion with the retinal image of other eye.

The long continued use of contact lenses can produce complications such as:

1. Changes in the curvature of the cornea.
2. Corneal warpage with increased astigmatism.
3. Corneal vascularisation due to interference with corneal respiration.

The recent soft hydrophilic (water-retentive) lens has been developed to overcome these complications, but soft lenses have other disadvantages such as the absorption of eyedrop and other materials, a liability to become infective, and fairly rapid degradation, which shortens their useful 'life'.

COMMUNITY OPHTHALMIC NURSING

Although there is a tendency for hospitals and their departments to become institutionalised, they are essentially produced and maintained by the community and should therefore serve the community as comprehensively as possible. In a speciality such as ophthalmology the patient often seeks specialist advice and care early, and much of the work involved in ophthalmic practice is concentrated in hospitals and specialist clinics rather than at the so-called primary care level. This may lead to excessive travelling for the patients, which is especially undesirable for those who are elderly, chronically sick, or recently discharged from hospital. The ophthalmic nursing service can be diffused out to the community in order to reduce this problem and a community service seeks to offer:

1. Specialist nursing aftercare for patients recently discharged from hospital.
2. Specialist nursing care for those patients attending clinics and who would otherwise require admission for treatment.
3. A diffusion of nursing skills and experience to those nurses unskilled in ophthalmology and practising in the community.
4. A communication link between the public and the hospital and a presence in the community, through the appointment of a liaising ophthalmic nurse.

The achievement of these aims depends on the nurses having a joint responsibility for patients in and out of hospital, and this requires co-ordination at a high level of management. Some hospitals maintain a 24-hour communication centre for enquiries from the public regarding possible eye symptoms and complaints, which need explanations and possibly attention by the doctor or by the casualty service. A diffusion of such nursing skills and knowledge into the community offers a better service and also a reduction in the demand for the inpatient facility.

CARE OF THE BLIND AND PARTIALLY SIGHTED

Such is the complexity of the visual process that the visual handicap can be extremely varied and it should not be forgotten that the 'colour blind', who merit no special favours, suffer a considerable handicap in a colour orientated society.

It is convenient that vision is assessed by fairly standard tests such as the Snellen's test type and the visual field tests. The complexity of the visual process means that the visual handicap can vary enormously within the same range of visual standards. For example:

1. *Cataract* often affects the distance vision more than reading and also can produce excessive dazzling.

2. *Macular degeneration* distorts the vision and usually disturbs reading more than distance vision. A complete central scotoma may eventually prevent recognition of faces and yet the peripheral field allows the patient mobility.

3. *Homonymous hemianopia* due to a posterior cerebral stroke will divide the field and may prevent continuity of reading across the page even when central acuity is perfect.

4. Peripheral field loss, as in *retinitis pigmentosa* and advanced *glaucoma*, will reduce the mobility of the patient, who tends to walk into unobserved tables, lamp-posts, etc.

5. Total visual loss, as may follow bilateral retinal artery occlusion

in *temporal arteritis*, will lead to a severe handicap, but may be accompanied by visual hallucinations, which give the patient a false hope that they still have some eyesight.

The recently blind need to be educated to accept their handicap and to use such vision as remains and to be helped to adapt through their other senses. The nurse, through an understanding of the handicap, is well placed to explain to the patient and help him overcome problems as they arise, although elderly patients often find great difficulty in adaptation. Many patients suffer great anxiety because they think that their visual handicap is necessarily going to get worse, and it is important that the ophthalmologist is told of these anxieties so that he knows of them when he explains the nature of the disease and its prognosis to the patient. The ophthalmologist has, in the United Kingdom, a statutory duty to register the patient blind or partially-sighted using a form BD.8; the nurse should be familiar with the structure of this form as it divides the information required into the medical and the sociological, educational, and occupational aspects of the handicap. The medical social worker can give valuable advice to these patients in regard to retraining and future occupational choices.

Nursing of blind patients is always a challenge to the good nurse, who will realise that normal communication is by gesture and facial appearance as well as by voice. The tone of voice often reveals the emotion or sincerity of the speaker to a blind person. It is important to reveal oneself by voice well away from the bedside; never creep up to the bed and suddenly startle the patient. Blind adults are adult and need some sympathy, but do not wish to be treated as dependent children. As in other nursing situations, the nurse may be guided by an imaginative understanding of what it might be like if she were the patient.

In Britain persons registered as blind become eligible to increased tax allowances as well as larger supplementary pensions and benefits. Assessment will be made through the social services in regard to educational needs, whether Braille or Moon alphabet requires to be taught and whether various types of occupational training are required. Many of these services are organised in co-operation with the Royal National Institute for the Blind (224 Great Portland Street, London, W.1). A minority of blind patients can be helped by guide dogs, which can greatly increase their mobility (Guide Dogs for the Blind Association, 113 Uxbridge Road, London, W.5). Partially sighted persons may be helped by optical low-visual aids which magnify, and are available through the consultant ophthalmologists' clinics.

The nurse should be able to understand the principal ways in which a patient with a visual handicap may be helped towards independent living; the social worker and occupational therapist can also assist the patient not only during hospital treatment but also after discharge and until the patient has attained his former independent way of life.

1. *Social work* is concerned with assessing the patient's disability in relation to his social and family needs, which are often mainly financial. The social worker will know to what government and other grants the patient is entitled and to what agencies the patient need apply for help with retraining for a job or other material needs.

2. *Occupational therapy* is not just a method of keeping a ward-patient happy and occupied with craftwork. The occupational therapist is a trained professional to whom patients should be referred for help and rehabilitation for visual and other disabilities arising from the long-term effects of disease and its treatment. Occupational therapy will include an accurate assessment of the degree and type of handicap together with its effect on the patient's cognitive, emotional, and practical aspects of daily life.

Rehabilitation will require the greatest improvement in the visual function possible, but may also require adaptation of the patient's home or occupation to enable the patient to continue independent living. This will require assessment in the home or at work as well as in the clinic, and the occupational therapist should advise in the provision of such aids as may be required, for example:

1. Visual aids – the best spectacle correction;
   low visual aids.
2. Mobility aids – walking canes, sticks, or frames;
   long-canes for extending sensory area;
   stair and banister rails.
3. Domestic aids – kitchen, living room, bathroom toilet and
   bedroom assessment;
   assessment of sources of illumination (window
   and artifical).

In the hospital environment patients receive almost total support for every aspect of living and the success of their treatment may in the end depend on a sufficient degree of support being maintained during their recovery from disease or hospital treatment after they have been discharged home.

6

Ophthalmic day unit

Organisation of unit
Admission procedures
Pre-admission investigations
Nursing care in minor eye
investigations, treatment and surgery
Removal of sutures

ORGANISATION OF UNIT

Not all hospitals have a day unit, but there has been an increase in these units in the last decade. The reasons are partly technical: the need to investigate more intensively or to provide a full range of care for minor surgery, but also social: the increasing number of nurses only available during the usually accepted working hours and the increasing cost of patient care. These units are usually organised with a five-day nursing cover and as the patients do not stay overnight, the throughput of patients must be well regulated. The administrative load is therefore considerable and the day-ward should have a large and pleasant reception area with a desk and records store closely integrated with the hospital records and admissions department (Fig. 6.1).

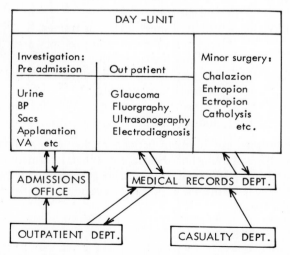

Fig. 6.1 Day-unit, a scheme showing relation to medical records and admissions

In those hospitals without a day unit the ophthalmic procedures described in this chapter are performed either through the outpatient treatment area or by admission to the inpatient ward. The day unit is a useful intermediate system for the management of these minor ophthalmic requirements; its success will depend on the bringing together of all the necessary hospital staff (doctors, nurses, auxilliary staff) and the patient within a fairly rigid timetable and forward planning is required if a breakdown is to be avoided. It is convenient if the structure of the day unit is located adjacent to the necessary surgical and diagnostic services and within easy communication with records and medical staff.

ADMISSION PROCEDURES

The day unit will be responsible for the admission and discharge of patients on a day-basis, therefore the record system must be efficient and tightly scheduled. Some patients (particularly ambulance users) tend to be late in attending hospital and a clear policy must be set up to preserve some flexibility for the reception of late-comers with sufficient deadlines, so that the work of the day unit is not paralysed by inefficient scheduling. This will be helped by the use of carefully designed stationery (Fig. 6.2) to include all necessary detail and the training of a co-ordinated nurse-care team on the unit.

The day unit may sometimes also be used as an admission filter for all 'cold' (waiting list) admissions, as the casualty is a filter for 'hot' (acute) admissions. If the reception area is sufficiently large, the expertise of the day unit in the organisation and admission of patients can be used so that patients with medical and ophthalmic disease contra-indicating surgery can be screened and referred for any necessary treatment before admission. A standard admission document may be helpful to standardise this procedure.

Admission procedures will vary, but should include:

1. Patient identification; hospital number, surname, prename, age, sex, date of birth, address, telephone number, occupation, general practitioner, social status (married, single, widow).
2. Disease identification: primary diagnosis, other diagnosis (laterality of each diagnosis).
3. Procedure identification: primary procedure (surgical or otherwise, for which patient is being admitted), other procedures performed previously.
4. Disability identification (functional loss which may affect nursing and medical care): primary symptoms, such as blindness, double

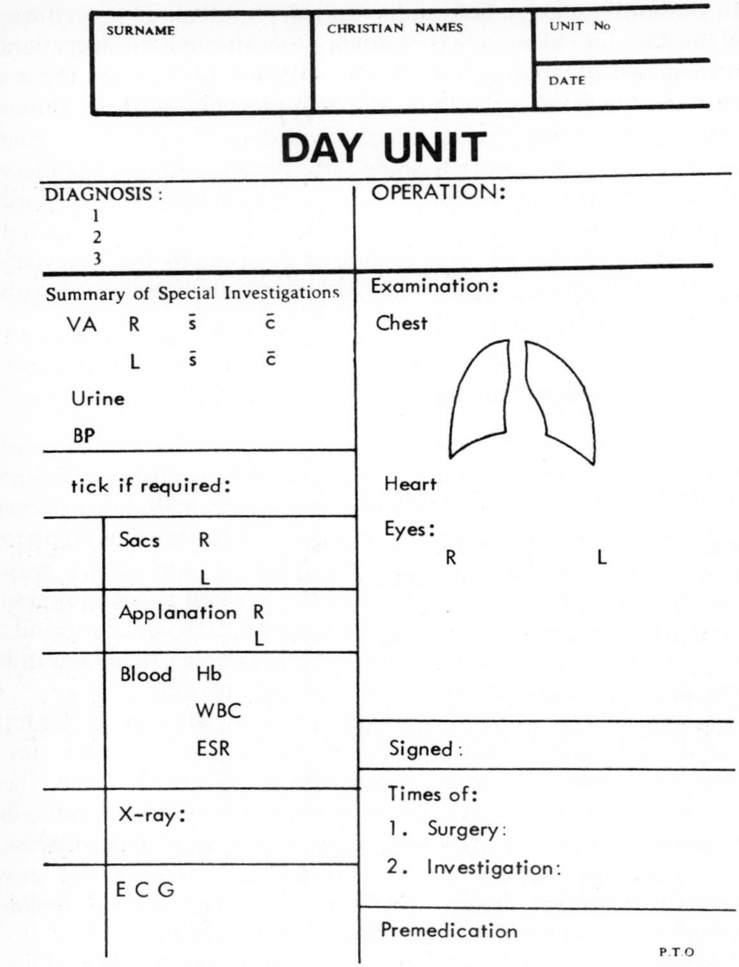

SURNAME	CHRISTIAN NAMES	UNIT No
		DATE

DAY UNIT

DIAGNOSIS :
1
2
3

OPERATION:

Summary of Special Investigations

VA   R   s̄   c̄

       L   s̄   c̄

Urine

BP

Examination:

Chest

tick if required:

	Sacs R	
	L	
	Applanation R	
	L	
	Blood Hb	
	WBC	
	ESR	
	X-ray:	
	E C G	

Heart

Eyes:
    R   L

Signed :

Times of:

1. Surgery:

2. Investigation:

Premedication

P.T.O

Fig. 6.2 Day-unit stationery

vision, watering of eye; secondary symptoms, such as backache, urinary frequency, incontinence; also any continuing treatment from general practitioner.

5. Examination of patient: visual acuity, urinalysis, blood pressure, external eye for significant disease or deformity, external appearance for evidence of infection or skin disease.

6. Identification of social needs related to treatment and aftercare. The unit will require a planned throughput and some patients with inadequate housing or no family may be unsuitable for day surgery.

Opportunity can here be made to explain to the patient the routines of the unit, the nature of his treatment, investigation or surgery and the planned aftercare. The nurse will naturally be receptive to the patient's questions and refer any beyond her expertise to the responsible doctor.

These procedures will be fully documented both for convenient communication to others in the unit and also for the medico-legal requirements for accurate records. The procedure should be completed by the necessary preparation for the duty-doctor's examination before surgery, and at this time a consent for surgery form (Fig. 6.3) should be available for signature by both patient and doctor. An electrocardiograph may be needed for patients with heart disease and some patients will require x-ray examination (chest, sinuses, etc).

PRE-ADMISSION INVESTIGATION

As intimated above, the organisation of the day unit can sometimes be extended to include the investigation of patients before admission as inpatients. This can avoid patients on the waiting list being admitted with a condition contra-indicating surgery. The procedure will be very similar to that outlined in the preceding section except that the examination of the patient may lead to referral for a second opinion on suspected cardiovascular or respiratory disease or further laboratory investigation and x-ray examination.

NURSING CARE FOR ROUTINE EYE INVESTIGATIONS

Nurses will participate in the preparation and performance of many investigations; the degree of their responsibility depends partly on their experience and expertise but also on the complexity of the task. Many of the routines described are also carried out in the treatment areas of a hospital outpatient clinic, especially when no day care unit is in use. Investigations often require the sending of specimens or documentation to other departments and the careful collection and handling of the former and accurate completion of the latter are both essential if the investigation is to provide useful clinical data.

1. *Lacrimal tests*

   a. Schirmer's test is a method of assessing the rate of lacrimal secretion, and is important in the diagnosis of 'dry eye', kerato-conjunctivitis sicca.

   The eye is examined for staining with rose bengal eyedrops,

WEST MIDLANDS REGIONAL HEALTH AUTHORITY

Wolverhampton Area Health Authority

Wolverhampton and Midland Counties Eye Infirmary

CONSENT BY PATIENT FOR OPERATIVE TREATMENT

I .... *of* ....

....

hereby consent to undergo the operation of *(1)...................... ....

....

the nature and intention of which have been explained to me by

Dr./Mr. ....

I also consent to such further or alternative operative measures as may be found to be necessary during the course of the operation and to the administration of a general. local or other anaesthetic for any of these purposes.

No assurance has been given to me that the operation will be performed by any particular surgeon.

Date............ .. ..   Signed........ ....
                                                                        (Patient)

I confirm that I have explained to the patient the nature and intention of this operation (through an interpreter) *(2)

Date........... ....   Signed...
                                                                        (Surgeon)

*(1) Specify side
*(2) Delete as necessary

Form 1   June, 1970

Fig. 6.3 Operation consent form

which are instilled into the upper fornix and spread over the eye by blinking. In 'dry eye' there is usually punctate staining. The excess fluid is now removed from each lower fornix with a clean absorbent tissue and a standard sterile strip of filter paper 35 mm long placed with one end in the fornix. The eyes are closed and the progress of the pink-staining lacrimal fluid examined as it is drawn along the strip by capillary attraction. The progress is measured after 5 to 10 minutes, by which time it should normally have progressed at least 20 mm.

b. Lacrimal sac syringing is used to assess the drainage of lacrimal fluid from the eye and obstruction to drainage often leads to epiphora. Successful syringing depends on a knowledge of the anatomy of naso-lacrimal drainage (Chapter 2) and a clear duct is signalled by the patient feeling the fluid in his nose or tasting the saline.

Tray or trolley

The following should be laid out on the tray or trolley: sterile pack containing syringe, lacrimal cannula, lacrimal dilator, and drawing-up needle; also an ampoule of sterile isotonic saline or other fluid if specified, as for example in radiography of the sac (dacryocystography).

The patient should recline on an operating chair or on the table with his head supported. Benoxinate or another local anaesthetic eyedrop is instilled into the conjunctival sac. The patient is asked to look up and back, the lower lid is gently and firmly retracted down with a finger to expose the lower lacrimal punctum. This is dilated by rotation of the lacrimal (punctum) dilator, which may be lubricated with sterile rectified paraffin or a soft eye ointment. The cannula and syringe filled with saline are picked up and the cannula gently inserted into the punctum (vertical to the lid margin), along the canaliculus (parallel to the lid margin), and into the sac. If the saline cannot be made to pass into the nose, the naso-lacrimal duct may sometimes be cleared by probing, but this is performed by a doctor, *not* the nurse; significant findings must be recorded in the patient's notes.

2. *Conjunctival investigations* are mainly to find an organism, which could be responsible for inflammatory disease, although many types of conjunctivitis and uveitis are allergic and not infective. As most culture media are very selective in the organism they will grow, it is essential to select the correct transport media on the basis of a provisional diagnosis.

a. Conjunctival swab

The principal requirement for a test: the sterile swab on a stick, and the swab is applied to the conjunctival surface. Contact is maintained for a few seconds so that conjunctival secretions may be absorbed into the swab. but care is taken to avoid contact with the skin. The swab is then transferred to the transport medium bottle and inserted deep into the medium, which will be of a type chosen to favour the growth of either aerobic or anaerobic microbes, viruses, chlamydia, or fungi. The transport medium must be carefully chosen for the suspected infection if the live organisms are to reach the laboratory for investigation. All specimens are accurately labelled and accompanied by the investigation request form, which will include the patient's details, the clinical condition, the side, and the requested investigation. In some units an incubator for culture plates may be available and the swab will be wiped lightly in a series of parallel lines across the surface of the medium, which is usually blood agar. Care must be taken not to contaminate the plate, which is covered and immediately placed into the incubator.

b. Conjunctival scrapings assist in the diagnosis of disease as they allow examination of the cells, which may be characteristic or contain intracellular organisms, as in trachoma and in gonococcal conjunctivitis. The requirements are: a conjunctival scraper (usually an aluminium rod hammered flat each end and autoclaved in a glass tube), a series of microscopic slides in a holder, anaesthetic drops, and sterile eye tissues.

The patient is laid on a couch or operating chair with head supported and the conjunctiva anaesthetised by the instillation of eyedrops such as amethocaine 0·5 per cent. The tarsal surface is exposed by eversion of the upper (see Fig. 4.9) and lower eyelids in turn and the scraper used gently but firmly enough to remove a surface scraping, which is spread on the glass slides. These slides are dried and sent to the laboratory for staining and examination. The mucoid scraping must be spread evenly and thinly, as the microscope cannot penetrate a darkly-staining globule. A combination of scraping and swabs for culture is often used, especially for trachoma and virus disease, but culture methods have become so reliable for ordinary microbes that a conjunctival swab alone is usually considered sufficient in the investigation of microbial conjunctivitis or for pre-operative microbiology.

3. *Blood Sampling.* A sample of the patient's blood is needed for many investigations such as an examination of the blood constituents (haemoglobin, red cells, white cells), the ESR (erythrocyte sedimentation rate), the blood groups (before transfusion) and the chemistry (sodium, potassium, chloride, urea, glucose, choles-terol, etc.). The blood may also contain evidence of specific infection (the organisms or their antibodies). The blood is easy to remove and has therefore become a useful source of knowledge regarding many of the internal processes of the human body. The requirements for the removal of blood from a vein include: a

sterile syringe of sufficient capacity for the sample needed, intravenous needle, skin cleansing swab, small adhesive dressing, compression cuff or quick-release tourniquet. The skin over the vein is cleaned and the tourniquet applied firmly but not too tightly round the arm above this area. The patient grips his hand into a fist until the vein dilates and the needle, attached to the syringe, is inserted bevel up through the skin and into the vein, following which a sufficient volume of blood is taken by drawing out the plunger. The tourniquet is loosened and the fist unclenched before the needle is withdrawn from the vein. Finally the point of insertion is protected by a small sterile adhesive dressing, which is kept on for about 12 hours.

Care is taken to discharge the correct quantity of blood into the container provided for the particular investigation requested. Some investigations require plain clotted blood, but when unclotted blood is needed, the volume of blood should match the quantity of anticoagulant in the container; the local information regarding the type of container and volume of blood should be posted up in the room where blood is collected.

NURSING PROCEDURES FOR MINOR EYE TREATMENTS

There are many minor eye treatments which are carried out by the nurse working in outpatients, a day-unit, or the wards.

1. Eyelid treatments include the epilation and elctrolysis of eyelashes, the strapping of an entropion, the trimming of lashes before surgery, and the use of hot and cold applications.

a. *Epilation* is the removal of an offending eyelash in trichiasis, when the lash turns inward to irritate the cornea. As the lashes are often very fine, illumination must be adequate, and some lashes can only be seen clearly using a slit-lamp microscope. The only other equipment needed is a sterile pair of epilation forceps. The eyelid is slightly everted in order to clear the lash away from the eye and the lash grasped with the epilation forceps. A quick firm pull of the lash along its axis should remove it out of the follicle with practically no discomfort. The removal of the lashes will produce instant relief of symptoms.

Unfortunately eyelashes grow again in about one month and as the deformity of the eyelid is usually chronic, relief is likely to be transitory; electrolysis offers a more permanent cure as the lash follicle is also destroyed.

b. *Electrolysis* (catholysis) requires the use of a small apparatus for producing an electric current, a cathode needle to pass into the follicle, an anode plate to contact the skin with electrode jelly, and epilation forceps. The eyelid is first anaesthetised with an injection of lignocaine, as the passage of current can be unpleasant. The anode plate is wetted with a small amount of jelly and applied to the skin on the forehead or arm, being either strapped on or held in place by the patient. The cathode needle, which should be extremely fine, is passed (under magnification) along the axis of the lash into the follicle and the current switched on low and increased to a few milliamperes, sufficient to produce frothing at the base of the lash. Once this has been achieved, the needle is removed, the elctricity switched off and the lash removed with the epilation forceps. If electrolysis has successfully destroyed the follicle, the eyelash will fall out without any resistance to the pull of the forceps. Many lashes can be dealt with this way, but if there is extensive trichiasis from distortion of the lid margin, plastic surgery to correct this distortion is usually preferable.

c. *Strapping for entropion.* A common type of entropion of the lower eyelid in older patients is senile entropion, which is usually cured by plastic surgery. Until this is carried out, relief from the trichiasis can be obtained by strapping the lower eyelid. A small centimetre square of adhesive strapping is rounded at the top and split up the bottom half. The upper edge is then pressed on to the skin close to the lid margin and the margin drawn down to produce a fold of skin before pressing the two lower tags on to the skin below this. This should result in a small degree of ectropion, and the result is tested by asking the patient to squeeze their lids. Ointment will loosen the strapping and must not be used.

d. *Trimming of eyelashes* is essential before most eye operations; if the lashes are cut during surgery they may carry infection into the wound. The patient should be reassured that the lashes will regrow in about one month. The following are required: blunt-tipped curved scissors, petroleum jelly, impregnated tulle, swabs, and receiver or other receptacle. The scissor blades are smeared with petroleum jelly so that the cut lashes adhere without falling into the eye. The patient is placed in a relaxed position with the head supported. The upper lid lashes are cut with the eye closed; the lower are cut with the eyes open, but the lid is drawn down and away from the eyeball, which should look up. The lashes need to be cut fairly short, about one millimetre. The scissors are wiped with the tulle between every cut in order to prevent an accumulation of lashes, which are removed before every cut.

Children will often be frightened, in which case trimming of eyelashes should be delayed till after induction of general anaesthesia.

e. *Hot applications* may be used to relieve pain or to promote the local circulation of blood in cases of local inflammation (stye, blepharitis, iritis, etc.). Traditionally hot-spoon bathing has been used and can be continued by the patient at home fairly safely after instruction. In hospital dry heat can be applied using an electrically heated pad or diathermy.

For hot-spoon bathing the following are required: a bowl holding at least one litre freshly boiled water, a wooden spoon padded with absorbent material bandaged over it, a waterproof cape, and a small bowl with sterile swabs with a receiver for the used swabs. The patient sits comfortably at the table with the bowl of steaming water in front of him and protected by the cape, which is tied around the neck. The patient is instructed to keep his eye closed and head well over the bowl. He then repeatedly lifts the spoon from the water towards the eye with the rounded side up; it should be emphasised that the steam is more beneficial that contact with the spoon. The treatment is continued for five to ten minutes and may be repeated two to four times a day. If drops or ointment are being used, these should usually be instilled before the hot-spooning as the heat will improve absorption of the active drugs; the prescription should be explicit on the order of treatment.

Hot-spoon bathing may not be possible for a child, in which case repeated hot fomentation can be applied to the closed eyelids; care must be taken that the heat is not too great as the fine skin of the lids is easily burnt.

A dry hot pad (Maddox pad) heated by electricity is a simple method and the heat can be controlled by a variable resistance control (rheostat). The electric elements are contained in a flat pad which is placed in the middle of an eyepad, and this is then bandaged on to the eye. The pad is heated through an electric flex controlled by a box containing the rheostat and switch. Mains voltage is potentially dangerous and the control box should contain an isolating transformer which steps down the voltage to a safe level. The flow of electricity is adjusted to produce a sensation of warmth and no more, as overheating can produce a burn and a patient must not be allowed to regulate the rheostat himself. The pad may be used for up to half an hour.

A hot water bottle made of rubber is sometimes used, but this should be only half-filled and should have two covers to prevent overheating. It is the duration of the treatment that is as important as the intensity of the heat.

Medical diathermy is produced by the tissues being placed within the field of high-intensity radio waves. This produces a heating of the tissues at a deeper level than is possible by other methods. The treatment needs accurate monitoring and is usually controlled by a physiotherapist with experience in ophthalmic treatment.

f. Cold applications are used to reduce congestion or arrest haemorrhage. Cold compresses using iced water or an iced poultice can be used. The treatment needs to be renewed at regular intervals, about every ten minutes.

NURSING PROCEDURES FOR MINOR EYE SURGERY

The range of procedures to be described are those commonly performed on outpatients or one-day-stay patients. Increasing hospital costs have created an economic pressure for performing more surgery on an outpatient or short-stay basis and the increasing safety of modern surgical techniques has made this possible. It must be emphasised just the same that all surgery can be potentially dangerous and the risks of each operation must be explained to the patient. If the patient's social circumstances or housing facilities are less than adequate, a decision may be made to admit for an operation normally performed in the day unit. Minor eye surgery is usually confined to the superficial tissues of the eyelids, conjunctiva and cornea; techniques for performing major surgery, such as cataract extraction by phaco-emulsification, on a day-stay basis have been developed, but these are not by any means established routine methods at present. General anaesthesia with intubation may demand a longer post-operative stay, often overnight.

Anaesthesia is mainly local for minor surgery, except in the case of children. Local anaesthesia simplifies the pre-operative preparation and shortens the recovery period; children admitted for general anaesthesia should have nothing by mouth for four hours previously and should therefore be admitted at least four hours before operation. All patients will require pre-operative assessment as described in the section on admission procedures and a pre-operative medication will be prescribed by the doctor, who has examined the patient.

1. *Local anaesthetic* will consist of an injection of procaine or lignocaine (1 to 2 per cent) with or without added adrenalin, which improves haemostasis. The requirements are a syringe and needle, a drawing-up cannula, the anaesthetic solution in an ampoule or in a rubber-topped multidose bottle, skin swabs in a sterile bowl, and antiseptic skin solution, such as hibitane in propyl alcohol. The

anaesthetic is drawn up into the syringe by the operator and injected into the site of the operation, which has been previously prepared and cleaned using the antiseptic solution.

Operations involving the cornea or conjunctiva will require topical anaesthesia using amethocaine or benoxinate eyedrops; they are instilled in sufficient quantity within ten minutes of the operation.

2. *Eyelid surgery* includes the correction of deformities such as *entropion* and *ectropion*, the curettage of a *chalazion*, the excision of small tumours, and the operation of tarsorrhaphy, in which the cornea is protected by the fusion of the upper to the lower eyelid. The form of the eyelid is determined by the tarsal plate and operation for distortion or for repair of injuries to the eyelid will require careful suturing of this if further distortion is to be avoided. The equipment required for eyelid surgery will include:

a. Local anaesthetic unless a general anaesthetic is used.

b. Instruments for fixing the tissue such as an eyeguard, Meibomian clamp, entropion clamp and stay-sutures. Also fixation forceps with teeth; Lister's forceps include suture-holding ribs, which are useful when forming and tightening knots.

c. Instruments for dividing the tissues such as a scalpel (usually handle with disposable blade), sharp-pointed scissors, and sharp-edged Meibomian spoon.

d. Materials for reapposition of the tissues such as a needleholder, and black silk (5/0) with atraumatic needle; catgut or collagen sutures may be required for buried sutures.

e. Equipment for haemostasis includes a bowl of sterile swabs or sponges – their size will depend on the fineness of the surgical techniques, and mosquito haemostats.

f. Receiver or other receptacle for used and contaminated swabs and other materials.

All equipment will be laid out in a tidy and logical order on a tray covered by a sterile towel. The precise method will depend on the local clinical practice and also on how much equipment is provided from the CSSD (see Chapter 9), and nurses are advised to make full use of manufacturers' catalogues to check the identity and range of equipment available.

a. *Entropion surgery* varies with the aetiology:

(i) Spastic entropion is usually caused by an irritation of the cornea as in keratitis and is basically a blepharospasm. If the entropion and consequent trichiasis is preventing healing of the cornea, weakening of the orbicularis oculi muscle may be produced for a short time by injection of the facial nerve with lignocaine or more permanently by a lateral canthotomy, in which the skin and muscle overlying the lateral conjunctival fornix are divided.

(ii) Senile entropion is associated with an atonic flopping eyelid and surgery for this consists of either shortening orbicularis oculi as it passes over the lower margin of the inferior tarsal plate (Wheeler's operation) or shortening the tarsal plate itself by means of a small wedge excision (Fox's operation).

(iii) Adipose entropion occurs in young babies with buccal fat. It is common in bottle-fed babies but is transient and requires no treatment, the eyelashes being soft at this age.

(iv) Cicatricial entropion is caused by scar tissue and usually follows a conjunctival burn, although it is also common in chronic trachoma. The correction of the deformity usually depends on total excision of the scar tissue (cicatrix), but in trachoma a buckling operation, which bends the lash margin away from the eye, is often sufficient.

b. *Ectropion surgery* varies with its aetiology:

(i) Paralytic ectropion occurs with a paralysis of the facial nerve, e.g. a Bell's palsy. Exposure of the cornea can result in keratitis and perforation of the eye. The lower lid can usually be supported by a lateral tarsorrhaphy, in which there is a fusion of the lateral third of the upper and lower eyelids. The margins of the eyelid are excised in a manner to include the lash-growing follicles and the raw edges drawn together by sutures until they have healed.

(ii) Senile ectropion is due to a weakness of the eyelids so that constant rubbing draws the lower lids down and outward. There is epiphora as the lower lacrimal punctum is not placed in its normal position to collect tears; often the duct is blocked and this should be investigated by lacrimal syringing. The entropion is corrected by shortening the eyelid and this is usually achieved by various types of wedge excision of the full thickness of the eyelid (Kuhnt's operation). In the Dimmer-Kuhnt operation the eyelid is split so that the wedge in the tarsal plate may be placed in the centre of the lid and that in the skin at the lateral canthus.

(iii) Cicatricial ectropion usually results from burns of the skin over the eyelids, but it may also occur with some chronic skin diseases such as lupus. The correction of the deformity requires the excision of all scar tissue and its replacement by a skin graft, which limits the development of further scars.

c. *Curettage of chalazion* is a simple removal of the granulomatous material resulting from chronic inflammation of a Meibomian gland. After anaesthesia the eyelid is fixed in a Meibomian clamp with its ring round the chalazion on the tarsal surface. The clamp is tightened firmly enough to prevent bleeding and is then used to evert the lid; the chalazion is incised at right angles to the lid-margin and the contents curetted with a Meibomian spoon. Antibiotic eyedrops are instilled, the clamp removed, and an eyepad applied firmly enough to prevent bleeding. The patient is prescribed one week's course of topical antibiotic ointment and the condition almost always heals without complication.

d. *Excision of eyelid tumours* should be complete, as the diagnosis of malignity usually depends on their histological examination under a microscope.

Benign tumours are commonly papillomata and usually occur near the lid margin. Xanthelasmata are creamy-yellow plaques seen in the eyelid skin especially of the middle-aged; they are not neoplastic but are lipid deposits which call for excision on cosmetic grounds.

Malignant tumours include epithelioma and basal-cell carcinoma (rodent ulcer) which often occurs in the lower lid and may involve the lacrimal canaliculus.

Excision of tumours depends on their size and attachment to deeper structures:

(i) Small superficial tumours are removed by excision of the tumour and some skin, which is loose and mobile over the eyelids. Undermining of the edge allows the skin to be sutured satisfactorily with 5/0 and 6/0 atraumatic silk sutures.

(ii) Wedge resection of the eyelid is required for tumours which have involved and become attached to the tarsal plate.

(iii) Plastic surgery with skin grafting is required to cover those defects left by the excision of large tumours. Without adequate repair, the eyelid will not cover the cornea during blinking and exposure keratitis may occur.

e. *Tarsorrhaphy* is an operation required to protect the cornea, which otherwise might perforate and it produces a fusion of the upper to the lower eyelid. Exposure keratitis and keratitis due to loss of normal sensation (neuropathic keratitis) are the principal indications; both conditions will produce extensive punctate staining with rose bengal eyedrops. There are two types of tarsorrhaphy:

(i) Temporary tarsorrhaphies are for conditions which are expected eventually to resolve. It is important that the eventual division of the tarsorrhaphy leaves a smooth functional lid margin, and in this type of tarsorrhaphy no eyelid tissue is excised. The necessary raw surfaces are produced by splitting the lid margin and using a mattress suture to pull the lids together firmly enough to open the upper raw area against the lower. The suture is left in for two weeks. Ointments should NOT be used as they melt and prevent full healing.

(ii) Permanent tarsorrhaphies are for conditions of a permanent nature and are performed as described for paralytic ectropion above.

3. *Conjunctival surgery* includes the excision of small blemishes such as a *naevus*, a *concretion*, a *pinguecula* and neoplasms. Injuries limited to the conjunctiva, such as a small laceration, are easily repaired as the conjunctiva is elastic and, except near the limbus or tarsus, only loosely connected to the underlying tissues. As with the eyelid, careful apposition of the conjunctival edges is needed, but finer instruments and sutures are used. The equipment required for conjunctival surgery includes:

a. Local anaesthetic such as topical amethocaine or benoxinate eyedrops. This may be sufficient, but if not a subconjunctival injection of anaesthetic is also used.

b. Instruments for fixing the tissues include an eye speculum, which separates the eyelids and exposes the conjunctival sac; an eyelid retractor, used to retract or evert a lid in order to expose the conjunctival fornix; fixation forceps (such as Jayle's 2 in 1) finer than used for the eyelids; conjunctival (smooth) forceps.

c. Instruments for dividing the tissues will be mainly conjunctival (sharp-pointed) scissors; a scalpel may be needed to shave a lesion off the underlying sclera.

d. Sutures for reapposition will usually be 6/0 black silk with atraumatic needle, but a fine collagen suture may be used for apposition of the subconjunctival tissues.

e. Haemostasis of the conjunctiva is usually achieved by topical adrenalin drops; subconjunctival bleeding can be coagulated using a fine electric cautery.

f. Receiver for used swabs. Conjunctival swabs are about 5 mm diameter, made of alginate or cellulose and are provided in a small bowl.

All equipment is laid out on a tray covered by a sterile towel as for eyelid surgery.

(i) *Excision* of conjunctival blemishes is usually performed by lifting the lesion with fixation forceps and cutting across the base with scissors. The resulting conjunctival defect is closed with a few interrupted sutures. The lesion may, if required, be placed in a jar containing formol saline and sent for histological examination in the pathology laboratory. A pinguecula is usually close to the limbus and requires shaving off the underlying sclera with a scalpel. Concretions are small accumulations of conjunctival mucous and may be removed by pricking out with a sharp needle. Neoplasms require complete excision to prevent recurrence and should always be sent for histological diagnosis.

(ii) *Lacerations* of the conjunctiva are usually linear and can be reapposed using a continuous silk suture. The edges of the wound may require cleaning and the underlying sclera should be examined for injury.

4. *Corneal surgery* includes minor procedures such as removal of corneal foreign body, removal of corneal epithelium and cauterisation of corneal ulcer. Perforating lacerations of the cornea are not minor injuries and require admission for treatment.

a. *Corneal foreign bodies* are composed of a variety of materials but it is mainly the metallic particles acquired in industrial work that become embedded deeply in the stoma of the cornea. For removal, the eye should be anaesthetised with guttae amethocaine or benoxinate. A good focal light is required, and they may be removed as described previously (Chapter 4).

b. *Removal of corneal epithelium* may be required for multiple scattered superficial corneal foreign bodies. The eyelids are fixed with a speculum, the eye anaesthetised with amethocaine or benoxinate eyedrops, and the epithelium rubbed off using a small eye swab held in forceps or a mosquito haemostat. If Bowman's membrane remains intact, healing of the cornea should be rapid.

c. *Cauterisation* of corneal ulcers is used to promote the healing processes and to kill organisms, mainly herpes simplex, which are not sensitive to chemotherapy. Although chemical cauterisation using liquid phenol or iodine solution is the commonest method, heat cautery using the radiation from red hot cautery close to the cornea is still used at times (chauffage). For carbolisation the requirements include a corneal loupe or other magnification, a speculum, a container with a few drops of liquid phenol, sterile matchsticks which are more absorptive than orange sticks, sharpened at one end, sterile filterpaper triangles (1 cm edge), anaesthetic and rose bengal eyedrops, and antibiotic ointment. The cornea is anaesthetised and it is exposed using the speculum; it is stained with the rose bengal and dried using the paper triangles. The match sticks are dipped in phenol and the stained area of the corneal ulcer carefully painted with phenol. The painted area goes white and should cover the whole ulcer. Excess phenol should be avoided and any spillage immediately dried off with a filter paper triangle. Finally the cornea is dried, antibiotic (or IDU) ointment applied, and the speculum removed. An eyepad is sometimes prescribed, although dark glasses are usually preferred as the eyepad may retain infected secretions.

d. *Pterygium* is a condition in which a vascular pannus infiltrates the cornea from the medial limbus; it is common in patients from a hot dry climate. If it is unsightly or affects the vision it may be excised and if severe, a corneal graft is required. Simple excision requires a final scalpel for shaving off the superficial layers of the cornea back to the root of the pterygium at the limbus, and dissection is then continued with scissors to remove the degenerate episcleral tissue deep to the conjunctiva. The operator will need forceps with teeth (such as Jayle's or Lister's) to hold the pterygium and a fine suture (6/0 silk) to suture the exposed sclera to the remaining conjunctival rim. In some operations the pterygium is transplanted and the procedures vary. The operation is usually performed with local anaesthetic (lignocaine) injected under the conjunctiva and topical benoxinate to the cornea.

Apart from corneal cautery and removal of corneal foreign bodies, the above procedures will not normally be performed by a nurse. The description of each procedure is therefore only an outline but sufficient to allow the nurse to have an understanding of the surgery and to assist the surgeon as required.

REMOVAL OF SUTURES

The nurse is often asked to remove the sutures after the surgical wound has healed. As these sutures may be very fine and the knots small, the technique used in general surgery is often not applicable and a second method is also described.

The requirements for suture removal include sharp-pointed stitch scissors, a small blade on a scalpel handle, suture forceps fine enough for the sutures used, a speculum and lid retractor, bowl of swabs, sterile towel with hole for eye, and anaesthetic eyedrops. If the patient squeezes his eyelids a facial nerve block may be needed, but usually topical anaesthesia with amethocaine or benoxinate is sufficient.

Method 1. The free end of a suture above the knot is held with forceps to raise the knot and one point of the scissors is passed under the suture beneath the knot for cutting.

Method 2. The free end of a suture above the knot is held with the forceps to tense the suture, which is cut from below the knot, but this is from outside using the scalpel blade. This avoids inserting an instrument within the loop of the suture and is both easier and safer when very fine suture material has been used.

Following removal of the sutures any treatment prescribed can be instilled. The wound should be examined to make sure healing is complete and the wound closed.

7

Inpatient ophthalmic nursing

Organisation and management of ward
Admission procedures and consent
forms
Nursing of medical patients
Nursing of surgical patients
Discharge procedures
Drug control

ORGANISATION AND MANAGEMENT OF WARD

The ward interfaces with the casualty and outpatients departments, from which it receives patients, and with the operating theatre and investigative departments, to which patients may be sent during their stay. The nursing staff in charge of the ward will be responsible not only for the continuity of the ophthalmic treatments but also for the whole care of the patient, who is temporarily a guest of the hospital and entitled to both physical and psychological support. The nurse is assisted in these functions by the modern management structure of hospitals, which include hotel, domestic and catering services as well as administration, pharmacy, and paramedical (orthoptist, physiotherapist, occupational therapist, radiotherapist, etc.). All these may require entry to the ward to perform their duties and the nurse-in-charge must ensure that such access is limited to times which do not interfere with patient care. There has been a move to recognise those duties which the nurse cannot perform herself, but the nurse may still be the initiator of effective action; all action must result eventually from individual action. There are many aspects of the ward environment which may affect the recovery of patients, such as:

1. Ventilation should be sufficient to maintain clean smokeless air, without chilling the patient.

2. Heating must be sufficient for patient comfort but excess heat will lead to sweating, humidity around the eyes and an increased risk of infection.

3. Cleaning of the ward must be effective; paintwork and flooring gradually deteriorate and redecoration should be arranged before cleaning becomes impossible.

4. Noise can be irritating to patients resting or with limited vision; sources of noise should be eliminated or reduced.

5. Beds vary in type and the type chosen must be suitable for the

patient nursed. A bed that breaks (that is a bed with a sectional mattress which can be hinged and inclined for greater comfort) can be more comfortable for a recumbent patient, and tall patients require special beds, a few of which need to be available.

6. Food must be appetising, hot as required, and nutritive; food is often a cause of complaints and these should be conveyed to the catering staff.

7. Light is particularly important to eye patients; some require extra light in order to read or for other recreations, while others with painful eye conditions require limited or dim light. Lights should, when possible, be controlled by dimmer switches.

The nurse cannot possibly attend to all these matters herself but she can initiate action to the relevant services. It is the ward nurse's responsibility to maintain high standards of patient-care and she can expect full support from the administration and other support services. Personal and immediate communication of problems is often needed if these are to be corrected; some, such as complaints about food or noise, lose significance as they pass into history, but others, such as redecoration and repairs, are long term and will need formal and written requests for action.

The organisation of the wards will be determined by the accommodation available, by the needs of the patient and the services. The needs of patients with eye diseases are usually most efficiently met by separate ophthalmic wards, but within these wards there should be a structural organisation to separate surgical from non-surgical cases or at least to segregate patients with infectious disease from those undergoing clean surgery. This will require an admission procedure, as described later, which recognises these differences. Some of the needs of inpatients have been mentioned; the particular needs for patients on an ophthalmic ward will include:

1. *A treatment room* within the ward complex. This will contain an area where ambulant patients can go for treatment, so that a comfortable adjustable chair under a focal light is essential. It will also contain facilities for the storage of dressing and drugs, including eyedrops. Sterilisation of equipment may be necessary where CSSD is not available and treatment trolleys, which go to the ward itself for the patients confined to bed, are prepared here.

2. *An examination room* is required where detailed examinations of the progress of the eye disease can be made by the doctors. It should contain at least a slit-lamp microscope with tonometer and visual acuity charts; a Bjerrum screen and indirect ophthalmoscope will often be useful.

3. *Toilet and lavatory accommodation* should be generous in space as

these patients may easily knock into one another or bump into a door jamb. At least one door should be wide enought to accommodate a wheel chair. Doors should not be secured from the inside. There should be no steps or other obstructions which could be hazardous. Floor covering should be easily cleansed, non-slip and non-inflammable.

4. *Bed spacing* in the ward should be sufficient to allow easy access to both sides of the patient for the examination and treatment of either eye. Bed curtains provide an easy method of providing privacy and also can help control the light during examination of the eye; the curtains should be of fire resistant material and should be hung sufficiently wide of the bed so that access is not impaired.

5. *Day rooms* are essential for the rest and relaxation of patients in comfort and also, by removing them from the bedside, allow for easier and more efficient cleaning of the ward. Here the patients can be provided with facilities for eating, television, and occupational therapy; chairs should be varied to suit the patient and should include some specifically designed for geriatric patients, as many ophthalmic patients are over 70 years old. For children the day room needs to be equipped as a play area with suitable toys, blackboard, and an easily cleaned floor, on which the children can play.

6. *Security* is required even though patients should be advised to bring the minimum of possessions to hospital, and certainly no valuables. Clothing lockers require to be conveniently placed to the area where patients dress and should be easy to lock and unlock. The nurse should be aware of the hospital authority policy relating to all possessions and valuables.

7. *Fire* is an extreme but ever present hazard and ward staff must be made aware of the fire alarm procedures, and use of smoke doors, exits, and fire equipment. Nurses require to be practised in the removal of visually handicapped patients, who are often aged, from the area of hazard and lectures and drill should be organised for all new staff.

8. *General nursing care* is often required, as many patients admitted for ophthalmic treatment and surgery have other diseases. The drug cupboard should contain a comprehensive range of treatments, which will be added to by the pharmacy on prescription or by a daily topping up system. A variety of dressings for non-ophthalmic use is required, and in older patients skin care and the prevention of bed sores is particularly important. Sphincter control is also often impaired in older patients and equipment required for incontinence and its control should be available, as well as facilities for hygienic disposal of all excreta.

9. *Visiting* should be considered in terms of the benefit to the patients. Visiting can be psychologically important in the support it gives and in maintaining family cohesion, but it must be regulated sufficiently to prevent interference with the normal working of the ward, especially during surgical lists, and to prevent cross-infection.

10. *A linen room or cupboard* is essential and this is usually topped up on a daily basis. It is important that regular checks are made to maintain an efficient service.

It is with the needs of patients such as these that the ward will be constituted and equipped and they will also form a foundation for the ward sister's management.

The management of an inpatient ward or complex of wards is a challenging discipline and though difficult, very rewarding in its successes. It will be appreciated that not only the patients, but also the staff, nurses and others, have needs. It should be clear that most nurses enter their profession with altruistic ideals of service to the community, and that the successful treatment of patients is a primary motivation which exceeds the details of contract, job description, or salary, and it is important that junior nurses are supported when, as is sometimes inevitable, treatments seem to fail and the patient's condition does not improve. The ward sister must also be aware that conditions outside the work in the hospital do cause frustration at times and the junior nurses often ask for off-duty to cope with these or with social commitments; one of the routine jobs which can produce many difficulties is the planning of the staff duty timetable, which must ensure the continuity of patient care. Nursing duties need to be timed in relation to the needs of the patients, the medical staff ward work, and the times when other staff, domestic and catering, etc. perform their duties on the ward. The ward sister will also require to maintain a high standard of clinical experience for student nurses, whose duties are arranged to ensure that this is comprehensive and covers the needs of the syllabus of training.

With so many hospital and clinical staff being involved in the practice and support of ward nursing, the sister will need to maintain:

1. A direct and personal communication with her junior staff and students through office meetings and individual supervision on the ward.
2. Telephone communication with support services will be required to implement immediate needs, such as the calls to medical staff, arrangements for follow-up appointments after discharge, and complaints regarding food and other services.
3. Documented records are essential on the patient's nursing notes to

provide continuity of care as these form a communication link between successive periods of staff duty. It is also important to document any problems which involve a delay such as a cross infection register and requests for repairs and supplies.

It must be obvious that the ward sister holds a key post in the health service and she will be responsible in the formation of policies of patient care and detailed planning, as described in Chapter 3.

ADMISSION PROCEDURES AND CONSENT FORMS

Admission procedures have been described in Chapter 6. It should be added here that the patient will come to the ward often having been on the waiting list for some time and he may have forgotten the details of treatment or surgery as described to him in outpatients. To relieve his anxiety it is important that he is received, as a guest, in a courteous and friendly manner and the nurse should make sure that he knows what his stay in hospital is for and what is likely to happen to him; also what help he is likely to require after discharge and how he can obtain further help (such as Social Services) while he recuperates. In most hospitals the patient now receives a booklet of general guidance before admission, but an ophthalmic patient may not have been able to read or understand it; the ophthalmic nurse should help him to do this as needed. Before surgery it is absolutely necessary that the site of operation is clearly identified by the surgeon, the patient identified (as with a bracelet) and the consent form (Fig. 7.1) signed and dated; any pre-anaesthetic medication should have been prescribed by a doctor.

NURSING OF MEDICAL PATIENTS

In ophthalmic wards all non-surgical patients have been classed as medical patients, although some of these will have injuries (such as hyphaema), for which no immediate surgery is advised but may eventually be required. This division from surgical cases has been made to reduce the risk of infection following intraocular operations, and segregation should be mainly on the principle of sufficient barriers to cross infection; manifestly infectious disease should be segregated further into suitable side wards, but the details of segregation depend mainly on the architecture of the ward complex.

Medical patients may be admitted for rest, observation, investigation, control of treatment, intensive therapy, and for segregation of infection.

1. *Rest* is important in concussive injury such as *hyphaema*, and is

WEST MIDLANDS REGIONAL HEALTH AUTHORITY.

Wolverhampton Area Health Authority

Wolverhampton and Midland Counties Eye Infirmary

CONSENT BY PATIENT FOR OPERATIVE TREATMENT

I .... of ....

....

hereby consent to undergo the operation of *(1) ....

....

the nature and intention of which have been explained to me by

Dr./Mr. ....•..

I also consent to such further or alternative operative measures as may be found to be necessary during the course of the operation and to the administration of a general, local or other anaesthetic for any of these purposes.

No assurance has been given to me that the operation will be performed by any particular surgeon.

Date.................................   Signed...
                                             (Patient)

I confirm that I have explained to the patient the nature and intention of this operation (through an interpreter) *(2)

Date.................................   Signed...
                                             (Surgeon)

*(1) Specify side
*(2) Delete as necessary

Form 1   June, 1970

Fig. 7.1 Operation consent form

aimed to reduce bleeding until the injured blood vessels have retracted and stopped leaking red cells. Haemorrhage into the anterior chamber or vitreous may also occur as a complication of diseases such as *diabetes mellitus* or *hypertension* and an initial period of bed rest is usually advised. Rest should be sufficient to allow for the correction of haemorrhage, but not so prolonged as to lead to general vascular stasis and a risk of thromboembolism. Physiotherapy with leg and foot exercises will help to achieve this in the adult patient, whereas a sedative drug (phenobarbitone, trimeprazine, etc.) may be required for children to achieve any rest at all.

2. *Observation* is essential for all patients and will vary with the condition. Patients will be admitted for observation when the disease is expected to undergo an acute alteration at any time or when continued observation is required to monitor the therapeutic control of the condition.

Examples include:

a. Temperature charting will be important in any infectious or pre-infectious disease.

b. Blood pressure charting is needed for patients with hypertensive retinopathy or with other vascular accidents due to hypertension.

c. Intra-ocular pressure charting to determine the diurnal variation of pressure in patients with suspected glaucoma.

d. Post-operative monitoring including a four-hourly TPR (temperature–pulse–respiration) chart when ordered. Post-operative infection may be indicated by a fever; blood loss and shock will lead to a faster pulse and respiration rate and a lower blood pressure.

3. *Investigations* may be carried out more completely and rapidly when the patient is on the ward, and it is important that the nursing staff ensure that the requested investigations are organised and completed as expected. Patients will be admitted for investigation if delay may lead to a deterioration in the disease. Examples will include:

a. Glaucoma in which an increase of intra-ocular pressure will lead to deteriorating field of vision. Glaucoma investigations, water-drinking test, tonography, etc. can all be completed and the patient's treatment stated and monitored within a few days, so that treatment can be determined and the intra-ocular pressure controlled medically or by surgery.

b. Uveitis patients are often admitted for rest and investigation. The aetiology of uveitis is often obscure, and may include systemic infections such as streptococcal, toxoplasmosis, tuberculosis, sarcoidosis, and toxocara, or an auto-immune reaction.

c. Neuro-ophthalomological symptoms often requre admission for investigation, especially if deterioration is likely or lumbar puncture for cerebrospinal fluid examination is required. Papilloedema and a history of transient blindness is almost pathognomic of a cerebral tumour and requires urgent attention.

d. Acute blindness is almost always an indication for admission and investigation unless the diagnosis is clear and treatment not required; this can happen when a patient with cataract notices the loss of vision 'acutely' at the moment he covers the other eye, rubs it, or closes it for some reason such as dust or irritation.

4. *Control of treatment* may be difficult to achieve in outpatients and a significant number fail to respond owing to an inability to instil eyedrops into their own conjunctival sacs. It is part of the inpatient investigation of glaucoma and uveitis to ascertain these difficulties and to train the patient in the instillation of eyedrops. In glaucoma treated by miotics such as pilocarpine, the degree of miosis will be a sufficient guide as to the patient's success in treating himself.

In glaucoma, diabetes, and hypertension, the potency of the drug and the dose requires regulation to produce control in terms of intra-ocular pressure, urine and blood glucose, and blood pressure respectively; this can be most conveniently achieved during a period of admission to the ward or sometimes on a day-stay basis.

5. *Intensive therapy* is required in acute conditions in order to control the disease and prevent loss of eyesight.

a. Acute angle-closure glaucoma is often associated with deteriorating vision and an intra-ocular pressure of above 50 mmHg. Medication to reduce the pressure will include an intensive application of miotic drops, usually pilocarpine 4 per cent, acetazolamide (Diamox) by injection and then tablets orally, and sometimes a diuretic such as glycerin by mouth or an intravenous infusion of urea. The intra-ocular pressure is monitored every two hours and after a sufficient reduction has been achieved, glaucoma surgery is carried out to prevent a recurrence.

b. Acute occlusion of the central retinal artery is usually due to an embolus and produces a catastrophic loss of vision for that eye. The resulting anoxia of the retina will lead to permanent blindness within minutes and every effort should be made to move the obstruction to circulation by lowering the intra-ocular pressure (paracentesis of the anterior chamber of the eye and intravenous urea). Vasodilating drugs have been tried, but not successfully. If there is a possibility of further emboli, anticoagulant drugs such as warfarin may be prescribed, but it is as important to ask a physician to investigate the origin of the embolus.

c. Uveitis can usually be controlled as an outpatient, but severe cases will require admission for intensive therapy, which may include systemic antibiotics, intramuscular injections of ACTH (adreno-corticotrophic hormone), subconjunctival injections of hydrocortisone, and anti-inflammatory drugs such as aspirin and oxyphenbutazone (Tanderil) in addition to the usual eyedrops and ointment. Secondary glaucoma will demand additional treatment such as acetazolamide (Diamox). Sympathetic ophthalmia, which follows injury to the other eye, is extremely serious and requires the most intensive therapy and supervision.

d. Acute optic atrophy due to poisons such as quinine (used to produce abortion) or, carbon monoxide (in coal gas and car exhausts) or methyl alcohol (in methylated spirit) require urgent treatment. Specific antidotes will be administered as ordered, but most of these poisons require intravenous infusion to encourage removal through the kidneys by diuresis; carbon monoxide poisoning can be alleviated by administering oxygen in high concentration to the patients in the inspired gases.

e. Injuries often require intensive therapy or urgent surgery. While perforations and lacerations of the tissues usually require surgical repair, other injuries, especially burns, require urgent treatment as described in Chapter 4. Hot metal burns may require the frequent instillation of eye ointment containing corticosteroids (hydrocortisone, betamethasone) with daily rodding of the conjunctival fornices to prevent the formation of symblepharon (adhesion of the eyelid to the eye). Chemical burns, having been intensively irrigated will need similar treatment although the formation of symblepharon is less likely. The insertion of a haptic contact lens is sometimes used to prevent the formation of adhesions but careful surveillance of the cornea is needed; involvement of the cornea directly through the burn or indirectly through ischaemia of the conjunctiva may lead to thinning and perforation of the cornea.

6. *Segregation of infection* may be required away from the family or within the hospital itself, and all patients requiring this level of segregation will be barrier-nursed.

Corneal infection due to *Pseudomonas pyocyaneous* is serious and often leads to perforation and panophthalmitis; it requires barrier-nursing and intensive treatment with a selected antibiotic such as thiosporin, gentamicin, or carbenicillin.

Keratitis due to adenovirus (ship-yard eye) is often epidemic and close surveillance of the patient and all toilet and treatment facilities is required.

Eye infection is a common result of systemic infections such as measles and smallpox; the latter was a significant cause of blindness in the nineteenth century. In these conditions the patient will naturally be segregated.

NURSING OF SURGICAL PATIENTS

The nursing of patients before and after a surgical operation requires strict controls which are not present in medical nursing. Once the epithelial surface of the tissues has been breached, the primary defence of the body is laid open to further trauma, blood loss, and invasion by pathogenic organisms. These considerations apply to all surgery but require special appraisal in ophthalmic surgery:

1. Further trauma may seem unlikely in an area as small as the eye and its adnexa, but the small and complex structures of the eye are easily destroyed by zealous surgery, inexpert overhandling, or by the dehydration occurring from the heat of the operating lamp. Microsurgery using finer instruments under the microscope was pioneered by ophthalmologists in order to reduce surgical trauma by greater surgical precision.

2. Blood loss is rarely a problem in eye surgery, where surgical precision is so important that even a small accumulation of blood impairs the surgeon's view of the operation. Operative techniques are therefore designed to control bleeding to the minimum loss, and this is especially important for operations which, like dacryocystorrhinostomy, involve the nasal mucosa, an extremely vascular area.

3. Pathogenic invasion leading to infection has been a major hazard of surgery since earliest times, and placed the greatest restriction on the use of surgical procedures. The development of antiseptic and aseptic techniques occurred during the last half of the nineteenth century through the application by Lister of the principles of microbiology formulated by Pasteur. The safety of modern surgery owes a debt to these pioneers; even though today antibiotics can be used to overcome infection, surgical healing and the results of surgery are almost always more satisfactory when infection has been prevented. This is especially true for a complex organ like the eye where surgical infection may be overcome by antibiotics sufficiently well to save the eye, but the vision is usually lost.

The prospect of ocular surgery can be terrifying to many patients unless the procedure is properly and accurately described; this should be remembered when the consent form is being completed and signed, and the nursing staff should at all times create a realistic level of confidence in the surgical procedure planned. In ophthalmic clinics when the surgical patients are segregated from the medical, the patient will inevitably gain some of his knowledge from the experience of other patients and especially those who have already had surgery; it is important that the nurse is aware of this type of knowledge and able to correct some of its exaggerations and distortions.

The preparation of patients for surgery has been outlined in Chapter 6, but the continuity of care required for the inpatient hinges on the needs of surgery which will be detailed in the next chapter. The organisation of a surgical ward requires some knowledge of the surgical operation so that the preparation and post-operative care may be planned. The details vary considerably for different hospitals, and operations; the patient's general condition, emotional needs, and social background should also be considered. There is a basic difference between intra-ocular and extra-ocular surgery based on the greater danger from infection for the eye than that for the adnexa; all the controls for micro-organisms and for the patient's liability to infection will be more detailed for intra-ocular surgery and should include:

1. Environmental factors in the patient's standard of hygiene, the cleanliness of the ward and the ambient temperature, which if high can cause sweating and moisture under an eye pad and consequent liability to infection.
2. Nutritional factors such as an unbalanced diet, a low or high body weight, pallor, a dry skin, or a smooth red tongue.
3. Systemic disease such as diabetes, which reduces the immune response to infection.
4. Signs of general infection such as pimples, skin ulcers, and paronychia (infection of the nail base).
5. Syringing of the lacrimal sacs to detect obstruction of the drainage passages with or without mucous or purulent regurgitation.
6. Conjuntival swab in transport media sent for culture and microbiological examination for pathogenic organisms.
7. Examination of the eyes and adnexa for any signs of inflammation, infection, trichiasis, or madarosis (loose or missing eyelashes).

Very many types of operation are performed and it is important to produce a procedure of patient care based on these principles, the needs of the patient, and a knowledge of the effect of surgery on him. For instance:

1. *Pre-operative care*
    a. Admission period to include documentation, identification of patient, type of surgery, and side of operation. Explanation to patient and relatives to include intention of surgery, visiting times, hospital amenities such as telephone, library, chaplains, etc.
    b. Preparation for surgery to include visual acuity, examination by nurse and by doctor, explanation and consent forms, checking of drugs, marking of skin on side of operation, checking identification bands, taking of culture swabs and sending to laboratory, urine testing, cutting of eyelashes, sac washout, skin preparation,

administration of pre-surgical and pre-anaesthetic medications as prescribed, and clothing patient as required.

c. Transport of patient to theatre to include checking sphincter functions, theatre clothing, transfer of patient to trolley and escorting to theatre while maintaining a reassuring confidence to the patient. The proper attention to theatre list times, and the identification of the patient when passing him into care of theatre staff.

The following typical check list may be used before leaving the ward:

a. Identiband is attached.
b. The patient is wearing a clean gown and that the operation site has been prepared and marked.
c. Male patients have been shaved facially and that female patients are not wearing coloured nail varnish or make up. Hair clips and jewellery should be removed.
d. The patient's bladder has been emptied.
e. Dentures are removed.
f. The time of administration of pre-medication.

The following information should be sent to theatre:

a. Consent form, duly signed, and patient's case notes.
b. Relevant x-rays and reports.
c. Laboratory reports.
d. Number of pints of blood cross-matched (when relevant).
e. Urinalysis – attached to front of case sheet, (especially when the patient is a diabetic).
f. Patient's body weight (especially children).
g. Any known allergies.
h. Any physical disabilities.
i. Record of premedication and other drugs and the time they were given.

The following points should be observed when collecting the patient from the theatre:

a. A senior ward nurse must collect the patient, and the theatre should be informed if there is a likelihood of delay in collecting the patient.
b. The ward nurse must check with the anaesthetist that the patient is fit to leave the theatre.
c. The patient should be in the lateral position on the trolley whenever possible, unless he is quite conscious.

d. Ensure that adequate information about the immediate post-operative care is contained in the case sheet such as posture, intravenous regime, sliding scale insulin instructions, oxygen therapy, post-operative drugs and treatments.

2. *Post-operative care*

a. Reception of the patient from the theatre to include identification, instruction from the theatre staff, care and escort to ward, transfer from trolley to bed and posturing in bed in accordance with instructions or usual needs. Continued observation of patient for signs of distress, pain or restlessness.

b. Care of recumbent patient during the first day after surgery will include continued observation, the administration of sedative or analgesic drugs as prescribed, maintenance of a comfortable post-surgical posture and the first dressing.

c. The first dressing is important and usually done during the first 24 hours. A sterile trolley is used with materials for removal of the dressing, cleansing the lid and lashes, observation of the eye with a hand torch, instillation of the eyedrops, and re-dressing the eye, if necessary, with eyepad and cartella. The doctor may do this, but if the nurse is trained or qualified to do the first dressing, she should report the condition of the eye to the doctor when he attends for his daily round.

d. Continued care of the patient will include regular dressing of the eye as frequently as prescribed, including the instillation of medication. Early ambulation is usual now that surgical techniques include adequate suturing with fine silk or polymer thread; ambulation improves the patient's circulation, reduces the weakening of prolonged recumbency, and helps in the natural use of the sphincters (anal and urinary). Continued observation of pressure areas and their care, and the use of toilet and hygiene procedure will be needed; the diet needs careful control in order to promote the healing processes. Patients (e.g. aphakic) may require the use of temporary spectacles after surgery.

e. Later care includes the ambulation of patients and adjustment to any altered visual function, such as the enlargement of objects and reduced field caused by aphakic spectacles. The patient will be educated in the need and use of post-operative medication, and in self help required after discharge, although the social condition should already be known to the ward staff. Operation sutures will be removed, if necessary, or arrangements made for this following discharge, and any outpatient or other discharge arrangements will be made, such as informing relatives, convalescent home, general practitioner, health visitors, community liaison officer and social services, etc.

3. *Special considerations for various types of surgery*

It must be emphasised that some knowledge of each condition is essential for the ophthalmic nurse, as can be learned from one of the textbooks referred to in the Bibliography.

a. Intraocular surgery includes cataract extraction, glaucoma surgery, corneal grafting (keratoplasty), and repair of perforating injuries of the eye. In these cases special care is required for the prevention of infection and the last will require a routine course of systemic antibiotic. Any pressure on the eye following surgery can strain and rupture the healing wound so that all dressings are completed with extreme delicacy and the eye protected by a cartella shield, which is placed so that its edge rests on, and therefore transfers pressure to, the skin over the bones of the face (malar, maxilla and frontal bones). As with all intra-ocular surgery attention to infection is especially important and may include a conjunctival swab for culture 48 hours before surgery, lacrimal syringing and trimming of the eyelashes. The patient is sometimes admitted 48 hours pre-operatively for preparation, but this practice varies and in an urban area with a premium on short-stay care many of these investigations are carried out in the day unit or in outpatients before admission. Some patients, such as those with diabetes or bronchitis, may require admission some days before surgery for assessment and control of their condition, and others require time to orientate themselves to the ward environments.

b. Cataract surgery is carried out when the opacity of the crystalline lens is sufficiently dense to prevent visual improvement with glasses. In younger children the lens usually is soft and can often be removed though a small aperture using a needle to break it up followed by irrigation and aspiration with a cannula and syringe or other suction apparatus. In babies it is usually impossible to keep a dressing over the eye, and it would tend to cause the child to rub this area with its hands; the eye is therefore not usually dressed though the child will require close observation, and sedation is prescribed in sufficient dose to prevent self-inflicted injury.

In adults the lens forms a hard nucleus, so that cataract extraction requires removal of the lens through an incision (the section) larger than the size of the nucleus (Fig. 7.2). This section is sutured with three to five fine sutures (8/0 silk or 10/0 polymer) and should be sufficiently secure for ambulation from the first day; leakage from

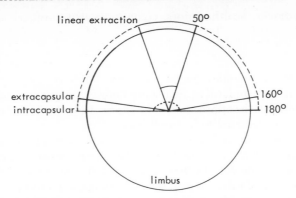

Fig. 7.2 Size of cataract section (incision) related to type of extraction

the wound will cause a shallow anterior chamber, which may require further bed rest and should be reported to the doctor.

Many cataract patients are over 70 years old and for these a local anaesthetic is often appropriate, and the premedication will include a hypnotic such as seconal (100 mg) with pethidine (100 mg) by mouth one hour before surgery. For general anaesthesia the premedication may include an analgesic such as pethidine with atropine intramuscularly. The atropine is important to prevent the slowing of the heart, which can be caused by reflex excitation of the vagus nerve through traction on the rectus muscles. Although any nurse care planning needs to take account of the local facilities available and the social and medical condition of the patient, the following procedure could be an average example:

Day	Procedure	Purpose
−10	Send for patient off waiting list	Admission of patient
	Inform general practitioner	History of recent disease and medication
−2	Admit to ward for:	
	1. Conjunctival swab	Exclude significant pathogens
	2. Syringe lacrimal sacs	Exclude lacrimal infections
	3. Visual acuity	Record for post operative comparisons
	4. History of recent complaints	Indication of recent disease
	sphincter control	Need for special nursing
	diet	Need for special diet
	sleep	Need for hypnotic drug
	5. Examination – eye	Indications of other eye disease
	– general	Indication of other diseases
	– x-ray & ecg	
	– blood pressure	Exclude hypertension
	– blood	Exclude abnormalities
	– urine	Exclude diabetes, albuminaria
	6. Eye treatment	Antibiotics to prevent infection

Day	Procedure	Purpose
	7. Other treatment	As required to maintain condition
	8. Explanation to patient	Reassure patient about need for surgery
	9. Explanation to relatives	Reassure relatives and explain visiting
	10. Consent form	Legal requirement before surgery
	11. Check prescription forms	Continuity of medication
	12. Check patient's understanding	
−1	Pre-operative preparation:	
	1. Cut lashes	Lashes impede access to operation
	2. Label side of operation (by doctor)	Prevent operation on wrong eye
	3. Doctor's examination	Eye condition, health of respiration and circulation particularly
	4. Check on operation premedication	Sedation before removal to theatre
	5. Check on patient's orientation	Ward routines often strange to patients
0	Day of operation:	
	1. Surgical clothing with split gown	Quickly removable clothing
	head-cap	To control hair away from eyes
	2. Dentures removed	Always for general anaesthetic (to prevent blockage of airway)
	3. Skin preparation	Antiseptic control of pathogens
	4. Administration of premedications	Sedative and analgesic
	5. Administration of eyedrops	Mydriasis improves access to cataract
	6. Transfer to theatre	Times by list and communication
	7. Escort to theatre	By nurse known to patient
	8. Reception from theatre	Recovery notified by theatre
	9. Transfer to ward bed	Extreme gentleness required
	10. Posture of patient	Recumbent but not too flat for comfort
	11. Sedation of patient ⎫	
	12. Analgesics ⎬	as required
	13. Continued surveillance ⎭	
+1	The eye will usually be covered by a pad and cartella	
	1. 1st Dressing –	
	removal of pad	Gently to prevent squeezing
	clean lids (saline)	Gently to unstick lid-margin
	examine eye (with hand torch)	For clear cornea, central pupil, normal anterior chamber
	instil fresh drops	As prescribed to prevent infection
	redress eye	Protection with cartella sometimes eyepad
	2. Ambulation of patient	According to condition of eye and suturing; it assists normal use of sphincters and the circulation

Day	Procedure	Purpose
	3. Explain to patient	Understanding of any restrictions
	4. Further treatments	As prescribed
+2	1. Dressing of eye	Treat as prescribed and also monitor progress – signs of infection, hypopyon; signs of injury, hyphaema, depth of anterior chamber, iris prolapse
	2. Continued ambulation and temporary spectacles	Circulatory stimulus +1O D lens for refocusing
+3 to +7	1. Continued nursing care	Includes treatments, diet, attending to toiletry, excretory functions, oral hygiene, pressure areas
	2. Explanation on post-discharge care Discharge procedure includes:	
	a. Prescription for further treatment	⎫ Continued care as ordered
	b. Letter to general practitioner	⎬ by doctor
	c. Outpatient arrangements	⎭
	d. Explanation of treatment and its instillation to patient and relatives	⎫ by nurse ⎬ ⎭
	e. Restrictions to normal activities such as stooping or hair-shampoo	
	f. Arrangements for transport	
	g. Inform admission clerk of ward vacancy	To ensure admission throughput

The schedule is approximate and can be altered or added to with experience.

c. Other types of intra-ocular surgery will require variations of care planned for each one, but the principles remain as for cataract:

(i) For glaucoma surgery the intra-ocular pressure will often be reduced before surgery by means of intensive pilocarpine eyedrops, diamox, or intravenous urea, etc. In the post-operative period excessive drainage may lead to a shallow or absent anterior chamber; a mydriatic may help to restore the anterior chamber by increasing the tension of the zonule (suspensory ligament) and stabilising the position of the crystalline lens. A hasty ambulation may precipitate a loss of the anterior chamber, as may straining during defaecation.

(ii) Pupil and capsule surgery is sometimes required following cataract operations. After an *extracapsular* operation, a thickened capsule may obscure the vision; capsulotomy using a Ziegler needle is a short operation which requires a very short convalescence even though all the usual pre-operative precautions against sepsis are still required. Following *intracapsular* surgery the pupil sometimes becomes adherent to the vitreous face producing a secondary glaucoma, or drawn upwards by the incarceration of vitreous in the section; in such cases the pupil can be expanded by either *photocoagulation* or by open surgery using iris scissors. Photocoagulation is a non-surgical procedure, but requires full local anaesthetic and immersion of the cornea by saline to prevent corneal heating.

(iii) Pseudophakos is the insertion into the eye of a plastic lens to replace the lens removed by cataract surgery. The nursing preparation and post-operative care is almost identical to that of cataract extraction. The patient should have a very much better vision than after simple cataract extraction and will find ambulation easier; an *aphakic* patient requires strong convex lenses and the consequent magnification upsets the judgment of distances, as mentioned above.

(iv) Keratoplasty (corneal graft) is performed by the trephining of the cornea and the replacement of the disc by a donor corneal disc of the same size and sutured into place. By this means corneal scarring can be removed and the vision improved (optical graft); also corneal disease may be excised and replaced by more normal tissues to assist healing (therapeutic graft). Nursing is very similar to that for a cataract, and ambulation is again started within a few days, largely due to the use of modern suturing techniques. For a penetrating graft, pilocarpine drops are usually prescribed as the miosed iris protects the lens.

(v) *Retinal detachment* surgery is aimed at flattening the retina against the choroid and sealing any holes and tears, which allow fluid to pass into the space deep to the retina. The preparation is similar to that of a cataract except that the patient is kept at rest in bed before surgery in order to prevent further detachment, especially of the macula, and to encourage some absorption of the subretinal fluid; for this purpose the head may be carefully postured according to the orders of the surgeon and lochbrilles prescribed (Fig. 7.3). The operation usually consists of some method of reducing the intra-ocular volume (by scleral resection, plombage, or encircling bands) and the production of a healing scar in the area of the hole by a choroidal inflammation (short-wave diathermy or kryopexy; see next chapter). So that healing may occur with the retina in the correct position, the patient is often rested for a few days, after surgery, but the use of increasingly precise surgery with accurate placement of the

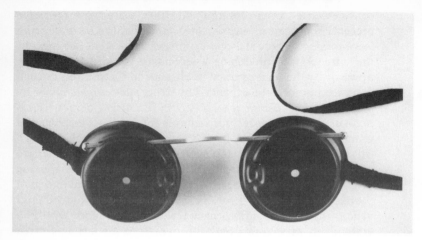

Fig. 7.3 Lochbrille

indenting plombage or band has made early ambulation safer than a few years ago, when prolonged bed rest in one position was the rule.

(vi) *Dacryocystorrhinostomy* is an operation for draining the lacrimal sac into the nose when there is either a chronic infection (*dacryocystitis*) or prolonged epiphora due to obstruction of the nasolacrimal duct below the sac (dacyrostenosis). This operation may be performed under local or general anaesthesia, but many anaesthetic gases dilate the arterioles and in an operation involving the nasal mucosa excessive haemorrhage can result and therefore it is essential for cross matching to have been completed prior to the operation. Control of haemorrhage is essential to the surgeon and the nose should be packed with a ribbon-gauge soaked in cocaine (10 per cent) and adrenaline (0·1 per cent) at least 30 minutes before surgery. If the operation is performed under local anaesthetic, the patient should be informed that a certain noise is inevitable from the excision of nasal bones. Post-operative care is aimed at the observation and prevention of any untoward bleeding and a half-hourly pulse is charted over the first twelve hours and the blood pressure should also be recorded and the patient warned not to blow his nose. After the day of surgery, ambulation is rapid though secondary haemorrhage should never be overlooked.

(vii) Extraocular operations do not involve any incision into the eyeball and include operations for squint and ptosis, deformities of the eyelids, and plastic repair for injuries to the adnexa. Sterile procedures and preparation are similar to those for intra-ocular surgery, but a pre-operative conjunctival swab for microbiology is not usual. Post-operative infection is not common, but when it does arise should be easily recognised and treated without delay. These procedures are almost always uncomplicated and rapid ambulation is the rule.

(viii) Enucleation is removal of the eye and evisceration removal of its contents, leaving the sclera in the orbit. Evisceration is almost only performed in cases of severe panophthalmitis. The loss of an eye is dreaded by most patients but often the eye has become blind and painful and the patient's general condition following enucleation is immediately improved. Enucleation is sometimes performed for malignant tumours (*melanoma* and *retinoblastomata*) or to prevent *sympathetic ophthalmia* from the injured eye, and for all these careful explanation is essential. In younger patients, a plastic implant may be buried and this gives the prosthesis (artificial eye) a more natural movement with the remaining eye. Preparation for surgery is as for extraocular operations, but usually eyelashes are not cut; this is because there is a tendency for the eyelids to overlap over an empty socket and short stubble-like lashes can irritate the inner surface of the lid. This can be prevented by the insertion of a glass shell in the socket at the end of operation. Often a firm pad and bandage are applied to control haemorrhage from the socket and the bandage should usually be kept in place until the first dressing the following day. Ambulation is early on the first day following surgery.

In order to carry out these procedures the nurse must have an interest in the surgery performed as, although access between the wards and operating theatre is regulated by the needs of asepsis, every opportunity should be taken to keep up to date on new techniques of surgery and to maintain a close professional partnership with the operating-room staff.

DISCHARGE PROCEDURES

After recovering from surgery the patient will need to go home and every care must be taken to ensure a continuation of post-operative healing without complication. Knowledge of home conditions is essential and all services required (home visits, community nursing, etc.) should be arranged. Relatives may need to be informed of the care required and on the use of any treatment prescribed. Outpatient follow-up and general practitioner care is organised and the admissions office informed as to the availability of beds.

DRUGS FOR INPATIENT CARE

There is a special chapter on ophthalmic drugs. Here it needs to be emphasised that the ward is an area where nurses are involved in the use of many drugs and proper care and procedures for their use and storage are required. The following instructions represent a basis for ward or clinic procedures involving drugs:

1. *Cupboards*
All medicines, poisons, controlled drugs, and lotions shall be stored in four cupboards:

a. Lotion cupboard for lotions and external applications not marked with special storage instructions.

b. Medicine cupboard for all medicines not marked with special storage instructions.

c. Poison cupboard for all Schedule One poisons and other substances which the pharmacist has labelled 'Store in Poison Cupboard'. Schedule One preparations for external use shall be stored on a different shelf from that for drugs for internal use.

d. Controlled drug cupboard – a small cupboard inside the poison cupboard containing only those drugs specified for control under the Misuse of Drugs Regulations.

2. *Keys*
All cupboards shall be kept locked.

Keys for the lotion and medicine cupboard shall be kept in a safe place chosen by the nurse in charge of the ward or department.

Keys for opening poison and controlled-drugs cupboards shall be held by the qualified nurse or midwife (state registered nurse, state enrolled nurse with at least three year's post-enrolment experience with the administration of drugs, registered mental nurse, state certified midwife) in charge of the ward or clinic.

All keys should be clearly labelled.

3. *Supervision of cupboards*
The cleaning and tidying of all the drug cupboards shall be supervised by the qualified nurse or midwife in charge of the ward or clinic, and the stock drugs will be checked as they are returned to the cupboard. Stock preparations may be topped up by the pharmacy staff using request forms, which will be signed legibly by the nurse in charge (or

her deputy). Stock preparations specified in the Misuse of Drugs Regulations must be ordered in the special 'Controlled Drug Order Book' and signed for by the nurse in charge of the ward or clinic (a separate requisition is needed for each preparation).

Stocks of controlled drugs shall be checked at least once daily by the nurse in charge or her deputy, and this check recorded in the controlled drug book.

4. *Drug prescriptions*

a. No medicine or drug (except as in paragraph 4.b) shall be administered to a patient unless prescribed on the patient's treatment sheet by a qualified doctor (registered with the General Medical Council).

b. When urgent treatment is required through the patient's clinical condition, a verbal instruction for the administration of a drug may be accepted by a qualified nurse, who shall be satisfied about the identity of the doctor and must record the instruction on the patient's treatment sheet. The instruction must be endorsed in writing by the doctor within 24 hours. When the instruction is given over the telephone, the nurse shall write it down complete and in longhand and shall read it back to the doctor checking the name of the patient, the drug, and its dose; the drug shall be administered by the same nurse who wrote down the instruction.

c. If a prescription is ambiguous or cannot be read, the nurse must communicate with the doctor or his deputy before administering the treatment.

5. *Labels and containers*

a. If a label is damaged or cannot be easily read, no attempt shall be made to amend or replace the label; the container must be returned to the pharmacy.

b. No preparation shall be removed from a container unless for immediate use or administration.

c. Unused preparations must not be returned to the container but destroyed (Controlled drugs must be destroyed in the presence of a witness and the destruction recorded with two signatures in the Controlled Drug Register).

6. *Drugs on admission and discharge of patient*

a. When newly-admitted patients bring previous medication with them, the doctor shall be informed. All hospital treatment shall be prescribed by the hospital doctor and these drugs either returned to the patient's relatives or (with the patient's consent) transferred to the pharmacist.

b. When the patient is discharged (or dies) all drugs dispensed for his use shall be returned to the pharmacist, except for drugs prescribed for his use at home.

7. Borrowing of drugs

Drugs must not normally be borrowed from other wards or clinics, but shall be obtained from the pharmacist.

Only in emergency and with the consent of the nurse in charge may a drug be borrowed from other wards or clinics; these transactions shall be recorded in the ward diary.

8. Procedure for the administration of drugs

Qualified nurses and midwives shall be responsible for administration of all drugs; learners may only administer drugs under supervision.

The following types of preparations shall be checked by a second nurse or midwife (or doctor):

a. All injections (except some injections when given by a community nurse in the patient's home, e.g. insulin, modecate, depixol).

b. All drugs from the poison and medicine cupboards.

c. All drugs controlled by the Misuse of Drugs Regulations.

d. Addition to intravenous solutions may only be given by a doctor or a specially designated qualified nurse.

Regulations

a. The following procedure is used for all injections, medicines, and poisonous preparations:

(i) Read prescription carefully and compare with recordings on container.

(ii) Ask the person who is to check the drug to do the same.

(iii) Prepare the drug and re-read the prescription with the checker.

(iv) Take the drug together with the treatment sheet to the patient. Compare the patient's identity bracelet with the name on the treatment sheet (both nurses to do this).

(v) Ensure administration of drug.

(vi) Record the administration of the drug on the treatment sheet with the time given (rechecking the name and dose prescribed).

b. Controlled drugs shall be administered as follows:

(i) Read prescription carefully.

(ii) Remove the drug, in its container, from the cupboard and lock cupboard.

(iii) Compare prescription with recordings on container.

(iv) Witness to do the same.

(v) Prepare drug in presence of the witness, rechecking identity of drug and prescription.

(vi) Replace container in cupboard and relock cupboard.

(vii) Record the following details in the Controlled Drug Register:

> Date and time of administration.
>
> Surname and other names of patient.
>
> Dosage administered.
>
> Balance of stock.

(viii) Take the drug to the patient together with the treatment sheet and compare patient's identity bracelet with the name on the treatment sheet (both nurses to do this).

(ix) Administer the drug in the presence of the witness.

(x) Complete record in the Controlled Drug Register, adding the signatures of the persons giving and checking the drug.

(xi) Record the administration of the drug on the treatment sheet.

These procedures must be strictly followed, except that in an emergency the details may be entered in the book after the administration of the drug.

The Controlled Drug Register shall be put out when the nursing report is given at night and in the morning, so that all entries can be checked. The register should be checked whenever there is a change of nursing staff in charge of the ward or clinic: also when a ward is to be closed.

9. *Misuse of drugs regulations*

All nurses and midwives shall be familar with these regulations. Prescriptions for controlled drugs must:

a. be written in doctor's handwriting;

b. specify patient's name and address (or hospital number). The properly completed treatment sheets will be accepted by the pharmacy;

c. specify the form of prescription;

d. specify the dose of drug;

e. specify the concentration of drug (if necessary);

f. specify the quantity in words and numerals;

g. be signed by the doctor;

h. be dated by the doctor;
i. be in ink (or other indelible writing).

8

Ophthalmic theatre nursing

ORGANISATION AND MANAGEMENT OF EYE THEATRE

Although the operating theatre is part of a hospital, it is in many ways separated on account of the need to maintain a high standard of asepsis. Access is restricted to the essential staff and users, who are required to enter by the proper entrance and change into footwear and outer sterilised garments as supplied. A strict discipline is maintained as surgery represents a high level of technology, which seeks to achieve repair and healing through surgical trauma. All surgery has a potential for harm and the delicate procedures required in eye surgery require a particularly high standard of operative care, surgical accuracy and asepsis. Infection of the eye usually leads to blindness, if not to loss of the eye itself, and routines developed for theatre nursing and for the pre-operative preparation (described in the two preceding chapters) are aimed to prevent infection.

Although the theatre will be sited in an area adjacent to or conveniently near the surgical wards, the restrictions on entry and the intensive nature of the work make it very different from other aspects of ophthalmic nursing so that nurses who take up theatre work tend to develop their talents for this specialised work. This may lead to communication problems with the staff outside the theatre through a lack of mutual understanding, and it is therefore important that routine procedures ensure a continuity of care as the patient moves into and out of the theatre complex. Theatre work continues to place a heavy responsibility on the nurse in charge who is not only responsible for the immediate problems of supporting the anaesthetic and operative work but also the continued maintenance of equipment, the regular supply of materials and recycled packs (gowns, towels, etc.) and the disposal of waste or infected material. She is also responsible for the proper condition of the structure of the theatre complex and initiating necessary repairs; she will have the usual responsibilities for

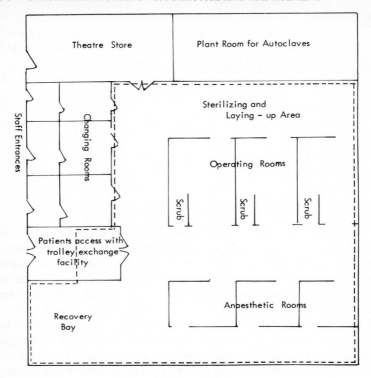

Fig. 8.1 Operating theatre, a scheme showing essential services

her staff, including their welfare, training and the maintenance of discipline.

The structure of the ophthalmic operating theatre (Fig. 8.1) will include the following details:

1. Access for patients, nursing and operating staff.
2. Access for the supply of equipment and sterile materials and for the separate disposal of waste and contaminated materials.
3. Access for service and maintenance, which is carried out as far as possible outside the actual operating area; this may be achieved by the use of a false ceiling and inner shell construction, so that plumbing, gas and power equipment and supplies are accessible on the outside of the shell.
4. Communication between theatre and the hospital will be mostly by telephone as movement of staff in and out is restricted to prevent contamination.

5. Ventilation of a theatre should be by a positive pressure supply of filtered air from a conditioning plant feeding into the operating area. Air movement is directed away from this area and all doors will therefore open outwards away from the operating rooms.

6. Water is used extensively for cleaning but undue splash is avoided as droplets contribute to the spread of infection and a high humidity makes the environment unpleasant for work. Toilet, scrubbing and cleaning facilities are kept as far from the operating area as is feasible.

7. Sterilisation of materials and equipment is sometimes carried out in a central sterile supply department (CSSD); much of the equipment used in an ophthalmic theatre is delicate and will require sterilisation in the unit itself; details are discussed in Chapter 9.

8. Illumination in a modern theatre is almost entirely by electric sources. Fluorescent light is an economical type of diffuse illumination, but for detailed surgery or other work a focal beam of light is needed; the shadow-free scialytic light used for general surgery is not suitable for the more detailed surgery and ophthalmic surgeons often use the focal source incorporated in the operating microscope.

9. Storage requires adequate space. Although the area of surgery is small, much of the surgical equipment (microscope, instrument trolleys, anaesthetic machine, giant magnet, theatre x-ray and other diagnostic equipment, etc.) is bulky and without storage space the operating room itself will become cluttered.

10. Patient support services will often be directed by the anaesthetist and include the equipment used in the anaesthetic room and recovery area together with an adequate stock of drugs for anaesthetic and physiological support. Emergency equipment will include cardiac monitor and defibrillator.

LAYING OUT OF INSTRUMENTS

The care of instruments, together with their laying out for each operation, forms a major part of the theatre nurse's work; many eye instruments are delicate and their care and maintenance is considered in the next chapter. The methods used in laying out instruments have changed in recent years with the availability of central sterile supply departments (CSSD) in many health services, although in principle this has only enabled the nursing staff to prepare for each type of operation several days ahead; the variety and complexity of surgery demands such a large volume of packs from the CSSD (with space for storage) that usually a compromise is made of those instruments and dressings sterilised in theatre and the more ordinary dressings, gowns, and other soft packs sterilised by the CSSD. Those eye units which have a sufficiently large surgical work-load may have a theatre sterile supply department (TSSD), which can be orientated to the specialised requirements of the theatre and by its proximity improve the recycling time of expensive instrumentation.

It will now be understood that although some instruments will be available in packs, even to the extent of a complete pack for each type of operation, and some instruments available direct from a steriliser such as the autoclave or hot-air oven, during the laying out of instruments it is the nurse's duty to make available to the surgeon all the equipment required for that operation. A glance at any surgical textbook (see Bibliography) will show the very diverse and evolving technology of surgical operations and it will be part of the nurse's duty to vary the laying out of instruments according to the surgeon's needs. The standardised approach of CSSD management is antithetical to this and the surgical list requires the support of a bank of reserve sterile instruments to be used to augment the standard instrument sets. There are so many instruments that can be used for each type of operation and a selection should be made according to the precise technique and the surgeon's preferences. Instruments should be laid on a stainless steel trolley which is clean and wiped with antiseptic; the sterile drape is separated from the trolley-top by an impervious non-slip sheet, which has also been autoclaved. The selection of instruments described below can be varied, but should be based on the requirements of each state of the operation so that no interruption to surgery occurs through lack of essential equipment.

1. *Cataract Set* (Fig. 8.2)

Item	*Purpose*
Swabs in bowl	
Receiver	for cleaning skin
Antiseptic solution	
Needleholder, Quarry-Silcock's	
Forceps, Lister's	
Forceps, 2 in 3	for fixation of eyelids
Mosquito haemostats (three)	and superior rectus
Serrefine	muscle
Atraumatic sutures	
(four 4/0 silk)	
Cataract knife, Lindsay Rea's	
Forceps, Barraquer's 11 to 12	for cataract section
Scissors, de Wecker's	
Forceps, iris, Barraquer's	for iridectomy
Needleholder, Barraquer's	
Forceps, Colibri	for suturing cataract-section
Atraumatic suture (one 8/0 silk)	

Item	Purpose
Cystotome	for cutting lens-capsule
Forceps, intracapsular (two)	for removing capsule in extracapsular operation; for grasping lens for intracapsular extraction
Hook, strabismus or lens expressor }	for controlling movement of lens
Iris repositors	for replacing iris into normal position
Forceps, tying Scissors, sharp pointed }	for tying knots and cutting 8/0 suture;
Syringe 5 ml with a–c cannula	for washing out anterior chamber
Eyedrops – atropine pilocarpine chloramphenical }	for instillation at end of operation
Sterile dressing (tulle) Eyepad Cartella shield }	for final dressing of eye and its protection

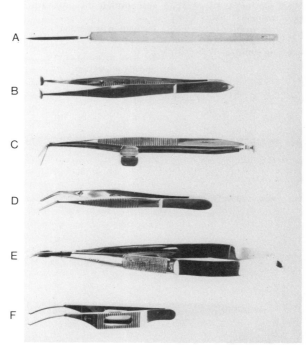

Fig. 8.2 Cataract surgery
   a. cataract knife
   b. forceps, fixation, Green
   c. scissors, de Wecker's
   d. forceps, iris, Arruga
   e. needle holder, Barraquer's
   f. forceps, Colibri

2. *Glaucoma Set* (Fig. 8.3)

Item	*Purpose*
Swabs in bowl	
Receiver	for cleaning skin
Antiseptic solution	
Speculum (right and left eye)	
Needleholder, Quarry-Silcock's	for exposure of eye and
Forceps, Lister's	fixation of superior rectus
Forceps, 2 in 3	muscle, etc.
Mosquito haemostat (one)	
Scissors, Stevens'	for dissection of conjunctival
Forceps, conjunctival	drainage flap
Knife, Tooke's	splitting of cornea in trephine operation
Knife, holder with scalpel blade	incision of limbus in iridencleisis
Forceps, Jayles'	or sclera for trabeculectomy
Trephine, corneo-scleral	for trephine
or	or
Knife, trabeculectomy	for trabeculectomy
Suture – 6/0 collagen	for replacement of flap and
Suture – 5/0 silk, black	reapposition of conjunctiva
Eyedrops – atropine	
pilocarpine	instillation as needed
chloramphenicol	
Sterile dressing (tulle)	for final dressing of eye
Eyepad	and its protection
Cartella	

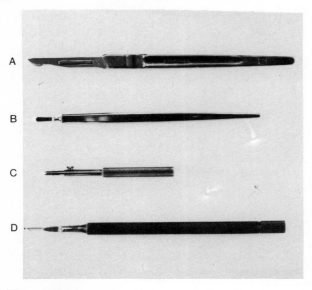

Fig. 8.3 Glaucoma surgery
  a. knife, scalpel blade
  b. knife, Tooke's
  c. trephine, corneoscleral
  d. knife, trabeculectomy

3. *Keratoplasty Set* (Fig. 8.4)

Item	Purpose
a. Donor Set	
Saline and antibiotic solution in bowls	
Donor eye in antibiotic solution	
Tudor Thomas stand	} for fixation of eye during
Sterile gauze	} trephine
Corneal trephine, Grieshaber	} for cutting corneal disk
Syringe with saline solution	} (to specified diameter)
Needleholder, Barraquer's	}
Forceps, Colibri	} for insertion of sutures
Atraumatic suture, 8/0 or 10/0	} into end of disc
Knife, Desmarres'	} for splitting of corneal disc
Forceps, Jayles'	} in lamellar keratoplasty
Glass receptacle	transfer of disc to other set
b. *Recipient Set* (Fig. 8.5)	
Swabs in bowl	}
Receiver	} for cleaning skin
Antiseptic solution	}
Needleholder, Quarry-Silcock's	}
Forceps, Lister	} for fixation of eyelids
Forceps, 2 in 3	} and of recti muscles
Mosquito haemostats (five)	}
Serrefines (two)	
Corneal trephine, Grieshaber (size determined by surgeon)	} for excision of diseased cornea
Scissors, corneal, right and left	}
Forceps, Colibri	}
Needleholder, Barraquer's	} for suturing graft in place
Suture, atraumatic 8/0 silk	}
Suture, atraumatic 10/0 perlon	}
Syringe with saline and cannula	for setting cornea
Syringe with sterile air and cannula	for reforming anterior chamber
Sterile dressing (tulle)	}
Eyepad	}
Cartella eyeshield	} for final dressing of eye
Eyedrops – mydriatic, miotic, antibiotic	} and its protection

4. *Squint Set* (Fig. 8.6)

Swabs in bowl	}
Receiver	} for cleaning skin
Antiseptic solution	}
Eye speculum, right or left Clarke's (adult or children's size)	} exposure of eye
Scissors, Bowman's or Stevens'	}
Forceps, conjunctival	} incision of conjunctiva
Hook, squint, Moorfields and Chavasse	} and exposure of muscle
Forceps, Prince's with catch	holding free muscle end
Caliper, Castoviejo's	}
Needleholder, Quarry-Silcock's	} measuring position of new muscle
Forceps, Lister's	} attachment and suturing muscle
Suture, atraumatic 4/0 catgut	}

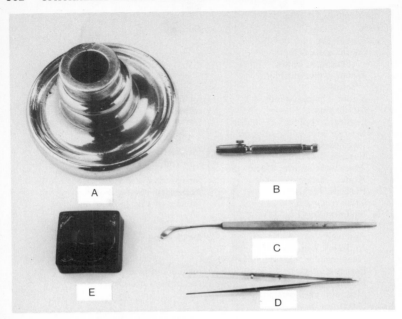

Fig. 8.4 Keratoplasty surgery (donor)
  a. stand, Tudor Thomas
  b. trephine, corneal
  c. knife, Desmarres'
  d. forceps, Jayle's
  e. glass receptacle

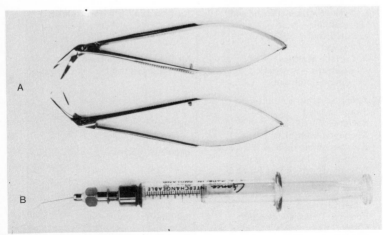

Fig. 8.5 Keratoplasty surgery (recipient)
  a. scissors, corneal, right and left
  b. syringe, air with cannula

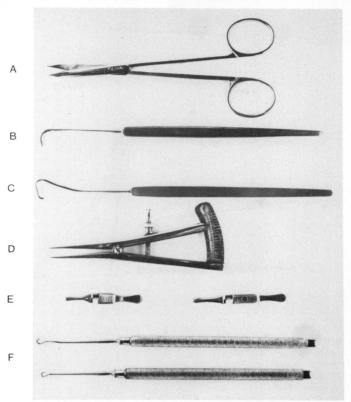

Fig. 8.6 Squint surgery
a. scissors, Stevens'
b. squint hook, Moorfields
c. squint hook, Chavasse
d. caliper, Castroviejo's
e. serrefines
f. conjunctival hooks

Item	*Purpose*
Hooks, conjunctival (two)	} suturing conjunctiva
Suture, atraumatic 5/0 silk	
Eyedrops, chloramphenicol	for instillation

5. *Dacryocystorhinostomy Set* (Fig. 8.7)

Bowl of swabs	
Antiseptic solution	} skin-cleansing
Receiver	
Scalpel, handle and blade	
Blunt dissector, Stallard's	
Periosteal elevator	} incision and dissection
Retractors, Bishop Harman's (two)	
Retractors, Rollet's (two)	

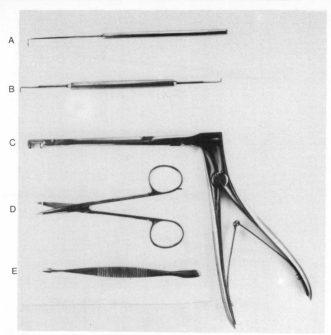

Fig. 8.7 Dacryocystorhinostomy
  a. needle, Dupuy–Dutemps
  b. periosteal elevator, Traquair's
  c. punch, Traquair's
  d. scissors, Werbs'
  e. blunt dissector, Stallard's

Item	Purpose
Dissector and Sac-retractor Traquair's	
Punch, Traquair's, upward cutting	fashioning of stoma through bone
Punch, Traquair's, downward cutting	
Punch, sphenoidal	
Dilator, lacrimal, Foster's	
Probes, lacrimal, Foster's	probing sac and fashioning
Knife, Hudson's	flaps in sac and nasal
Scissors, Werb's	
Forceps, Jayle's	
Needles, Dupuy-Dutemps' (right and left)	suturing posterior flaps
Forceps, Lister's	
Needleholder, Quarry-Silcock's	suturing anterior flaps
Suture, atraumatic 5/0 black silk	and skin
Skin-hooks, Kilner's (two)	

6. *Enucleation Set* (Fig. 8.8)

Bowls with swabs	
Antiseptic solution in bowl	skin cleansing
Receiver	

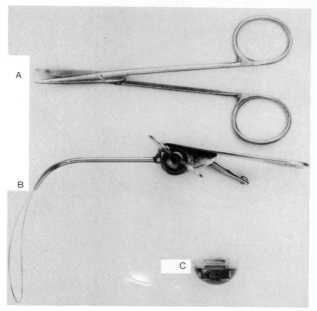

Fig. 8.8 Enucleation surgery
a. scissors, curved-on-flat
b. snare, Foster's
c. plastic implant, Roper-Hall

Item	*Purpose*
Eye speculum, Clarke's Scissors, conjunctival, sharp- points Forceps, conjunctival	dissection of conjunctiva
Scissors, squint, Stevens' Squint-hooks, Moorfield's Sutures, atraumatic, catgut, 4/0 Needleholder, Quarry-Silcock's Forceps, Lister's	dissection, and identification of muscles, suturing tendons to implant and closing conjunctival wound
Scissors, curved-on-flat, or Snare, enucleation, Foster's	cutting of optic nerve
Plastic implant, Allen's or Roper-Hall	replaces eye and enables muscles to move prosthesis
Suture, atraumatic, catgut, 4/0	closure of operation
Suture, atraumatic, silk, 5/0	wound

7. *Retinal Detachment Set* (Fig. 8.9)

Bowl of swabs Antiseptic solution Receiver	skin cleansing
Speculum – Clarke's rigid Scissors, conjunctival Forceps, conjunctival	exposure of eye and globe

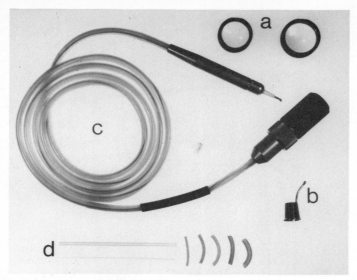

Fig. 8.9 Detachment surgery
  a. lens for ophthalmoscopy
  b. scleral depressor
  c. kryo–probe
  d. silastic sponge implants

Item	*Purpose*
Needleholder, Quarry-Silcock's	
Forceps, Lister's	dissection and holding of
Squint-hook, Moorfield's	rectus muscle, cutting
Suture, atraumatic, 4/0 silk (four)	insertion as needed
Suture, atraumatic, 4/0 catgut	
Scissors, Stevens'	
Haemostats, mosquito (three)	
Binocular ophthalmoscopic lens	
Scleral depressor	localisation of retinal
Kryoprobe	tear and kryopexy
Scalpel, holder and blade	
Needleholder, Barraquer's	fashioning scleral-bed
Forceps, Jayle's	and the fixation of
Silastic or sponge implant	scleral implant
Suture, atraumatic 4/0 polyamide	
Lacrimal dilator for drainage	
Suture, atraumatic, conjunctival, 5/0	suturing of conjunctiva
Eyedrops – atropine 1 per cent	and instillation of
chloramphenicol	eyedrops
0.5 per cent	
Eyepad, cartella, etc.	final dressing.

In practice the lists above will be seen to be a minimum requirement and a study of the actual requirement in each individual theatre leads to the addition of a reserve set and ground (or foundation) sets. A reserve set includes all those instruments that may be required by the surgeon according to the many variations of surgical technique and to allow flexibility in the operation without overloading the standard set. The ground set can be regarded as a set providing instruments common to a group of sets; for example:

1. An *extraocular set* should include instruments and equipment needed for skin-cleansing, suturing with the larger atraumatic sutures (3/0 to 5/0), scalpel (handle and blade), skin and squint scissors, antibiotic eyedrops, etc.

2. An *intraocular set* should include instruments and equipment for skin-cleansing, suturing with the smaller atraumatic sutures (6/0 to 10/0), iris scissors and forceps, miotic, mydriatic, and antibiotic eyedrops, etc.

The handling of instruments needs care as many are delicate and expensive. The traditional Cheadle's forceps has been displaced in favour of the 'clean' nurse wearing surgical gloves. Gloves are easily damaged and the nurse must be most careful not to touch any sharp part of the instrument and restrict handling to that part of the instrument handled by the surgeon, laying the instruments flat in such a way that the operative end does not (as far as possible) touch the tray-drape. The nurse requires to maintain the same 'no touch' technique as the surgeon, who also confines his handling of instruments to those parts which do not come in contact with the patient's tissues.

NURSING PROCEDURES (ANAESTHETIC)

The pre-operative care of the patient has been described in the previous chapter, and the care in theatre must be continuous with that, even though the conditions are different. The nurse who accompanies the patient to theatre should stay until the anaesthetist has induced the patient or, for local anaesthetic, instructed by the theatre superintendent; this nurse should continue friendly conversation, as required, with the patient, as well as informing the theatre staff about the pre-operative preparation of the patient.

The theatre nurse should check on the following details:

1. The identity of the patient by name against that on the operation list and on the identity-bracelet.
2. The type and side of operation as on the list and as specified in the patient's notes.
3. The pre-operative preparation as described in the notes and on the operation ward form; and confirmed by the ward-nurse.

4. The consent form in the patient's notes should be complete and signed by patient (or relative of minor) as well as surgeon.
5. Any prostheses worn by patient, such as dentures, contact lenses, artificial eye, should have been removed.
6. Blood is rarely needed for eye surgery, but if supplied identify by name, group, and hospital number on the label and patient's notes should be checked.

If the patient is to have a general anaesthetic the nurse should check the condition of the anaesthetic apparatus including all cylinders, all vapourising bottles, soda-lime in containers, suction apparatus, light sources including the laryngoscopes, and all anaesthetic drugs. In some theatres these duties are delegated to the theatre technician although the nurse-in-charge maintains a supervisory responsibility and should maintain all equipment in theatre in a completely reliable condition. Any recent defect should be reported to the anaesthetist. The nurse may also be instructed to draw up certain drugs into the syringe under the anaesthetist's supervision.

No patient can be completely comfortable on a theatre trolley but the nurse should make him as comfortable as circumstances and his anxieties allow. During the induction of the general anaesthetic the nurse shall help to position the patient's head and neck in the extended position required for laryngoscopy and intubation of the trachea as well as passing to the anaesthetist any equipment or drugs requested.

NURSING PROCEDURES (OPERATIVE)

Within the operation unit of the theatre the patient will often be under general anaesthetic; if a local anaesthetic is used pre-operative hypnotic drugs should be sufficient to allay anxiety. For some patients the latent fears of surgery only become manifest at this time and the comforting words of the nurse or the holding of the nurse's hand can do much to allay these fears.

The traditional ophthalmic operating table was flat with an adjustable head-rest. This type of table is not sufficiently comfortable for many patients, who may require a 'break' in the middle of the table to accommodate a curvature of the spine (kyphosis) and a tilt of the table to ease the respiration. The table needs to tilt head down (Trendelenburg) in cases of anaesthetic emergency such as the bronchial inhalation of vomit, or feet down (reversed Trendelenburg) to reduce the bleeding in operations such as dacryocystorrhinostomy, and a suitable table is illustrated (Fig. 8.10). The patient's head especially requires to be both comfortable and secure and a head rest

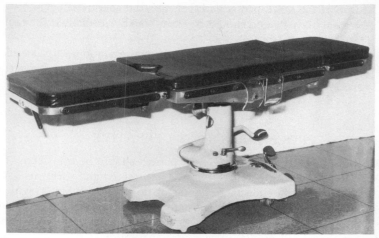

Fig. 8.10 Surgical operating table

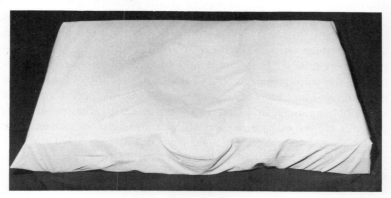

Fig. 8.11 Ruben headrest for surgery (with sterilised drape)

such as that in Fig. 8.11 can be used. Many attachments such as instrument trays, foot rests, and arm supports are supplied as accessories for the standard operating table and the nurse should be familiar with their use as well as expert in the adjustment and maintenance of the table itself. The patient is usually transferred from the trolley to the table on the same canvas stretcher that is used to convey him from the ward bed and back; all transferring procedures are hazardous and the condition of the canvas and its supporting rods should be inspected regularly.

The position of the patient on the table should be checked and the patient made comfortable. An unconscious patient is especially at risk and the following should be checked:

1. Support for head, arms, and feet must be adequate.
2. Natural body flexion should be maintained, especially if the table is tilted.
3. Support should encourage natural respiration, and no area should bear undue pressure which could restrict circulation or damage a nerve.

NURSING PROCEDURES (POST-OPERATIVE)

When the operation is complete the patient should be transferred to the trolley in a position agreed by the anaethetist and surgeon. The anaesthetist often requests a lateral position (such as Sim's) which ensures a clear airway, and it is usually preferable that the operated eye should be above the unoperated. After retinal detachment surgery the patient's head may require a special position, which should be detailed by the surgeon and written in the patient's notes.

The post-operative care should extend to the time that the patient leaves theatre and this should not be before both the surgeon and anaesthetist are satisfied that he is sufficiently recovered. During this period a regular observation should be kept of the patient's skin colour, the respiration rate and character and of the pulse rate and character. The recovery area should be supplied with a sphygmomanometer and suction apparatus with catheters, and the patient's trolley with an oxygen cylinder and mask or catheter; the trolley should be able to be tilted head down (Fig. 8.12) and side supports should hinge up to prevent the patient falling. The following complications may occur:

1. *Cyanosis* is a darkening of the skin due to incomplete oxygenation of the blood. Respiration should be encouraged by placing the fingers behind the angle of the jaw and lifting the jaw up and extending the head; this lifts the relaxed tongue away from the pharynx.

2. *Vomiting* may lead to inhalation and respiratory obstruction. The patient's head should be immediately turned to the side and the patient placed in the lateral or Sim's position. Suction will be needed, the anaesthetist being informed.

3. *Shock* is unusual after eye surgery, as the total blood loss should be small; exceptional operations such as exenteration or dacryocystorrhinostomy may lead to significant blood loss. Shock is suggested by skin pallor, weak pulse, and falling blood pressure; treatment requires replacement of the blood-volume by transfusion and the surgeon should be notified immediately.

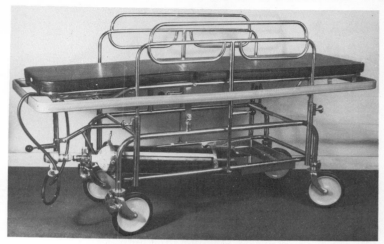

Fig. 8.12 Trolley – for transporting patient (note side guards)

4. *Restlessness and pain* may require the administration of post-operative medication (hypnotic or analgesic drugs).

5. *Cardiac Arrest* is a rare occurrence, but the theatre staff should always be fully prepared if treatment is to have any chance of success. The theatre staff should be trained in the use of the electrocardiograph oscilloscope, defibrillator, and resuscitation trolley. Cardiac arrest should be suspected if there is an acute apnoea, absence of pulse, mydriasis and progressive aganosis.

OPHTHALMIC SURGICAL INSTRUMENTS

Examination of ophthalmic instruments shows them to be on the whole lighter, more delicate, and more precise than those used in other types of surgery (except hand surgery, which makes use of some ophthalmic instruments such as Barraquer's needleholder). The instruments need to be used and treated with great care and the nurse should know the principles of ergonomics used in their design.

The *structure* of the instrument has two parts, the surgeon's and the patient's. The surgeon's part may be the simple handle of the scalpel, the ringed levers of scissors or the spring-loaded lever of a needleholder, forceps, or spring-scissors; it is through this part that the surgeon exerts his delicate and precise control on the instrument and the nurse should be aware of the differences in size, shape and surface texture which affect this control. An examination of the wide variety of instruments available will emphasise this as well as the

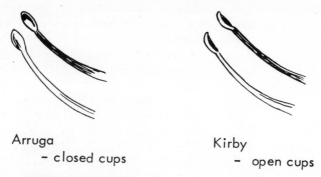

Arruga
— closed cups

Kirby
— open cups

Fig. 8.13 Comparison of tips of Arruga and Kirby forceps for intracapsular cataract surgery

personal needs of different surgeons, who will have anatomically different hands as well as basically different techniques in using the instruments. A single example may make it clearer: Fig. 8.13 shows two intracapsular forceps with almost identical tips, the Arruga and the Kirby. The Kirby forceps have a finer grooved surface, which may improve control by increasing friction between instrument and fingers, but also increases the number of crevices which can lodge particles of dirt. The Kirby instrument is cylindrical, which helps rotation between the finger and thumb, where as the flatter surface of Arruga forceps gives the finger and thumb a certain stability as well as a directional control through the sensation of the skin receptors.

The patient's part of the instrument is adapted to the surgical technique at each stage of the operation and this has been made clear in the sample lists of surgical equipment for the surgical sets. The comparison of instruments of a similar type make it clear that microsurgery has been made possible not only by using the operating microscope but also the manufacture of fine sutures with appropriate needles and a whole set of new instruments adapted for use with these finer materials. It is possible to ruin a small delicate needle with a larger type of needleholder and it is equally possible for the more delicate needleholders to be ruined if they are continually used to grip the larger surgical needles. Instruments need to be grouped into sets not only according to the operation but also the technique to be used.

The *material* of the instrument deserves some consideration although the majority are now made of stainless steel. Stainless steel wears well and the instrument stands up to repeated heat-sterilisation, but the alloy used consists of iron with the addition of chromium nickel, which softens the iron. Steel used to produce a sharp cutting edge cannot be soft and there is a limit to its stainless quality; some discoloration of cataract knives and trephines is therefore to be expected and should not alarm the nurse, although all such instruments should be sterilised dry, as in a hot air oven. The more stainless types of steel tend to be non-magnetic, and a special set of these can be obtained for use in magnetic removal of intraocular foreign bodies.

The suture needle now used is almost entirely the atraumatic stainless steel needle swaged on to a suture by the manufacturer and supplied in a sterilised packet. The older needle with eye was of tempered steel and therefore of the same quality throughout, but the atraumatic is only tempered towards the point, the other end being left, as soft untempered steel and hollowed for attachment to the suture; this part of the needle is easily distorted and bent and care must be taken that the needleholder grasps the atraumatic needle well away from the suture and about half way down the needle.

The material used for sutures needs to have tensile strength and flexibility, with a surface smooth enough to pass through the tissues easily but not so smooth as to enable the surgical knot to loosen or spontaneously become untied. Sutures are mostly composed of polymers, which may be natural (catgut, silk) or synthetic (polyglycolic acid, polyester). Stainless steel wire has not been used much in eye surgery but tantalum wire mesh is sometimes used in repair of the orbit. Acrylic polymer and siliconised latex are used in the manufacture of orbital implants and the former is used for pseudophakos (the lenticular implant, which sometimes replaces the crystalline-lens after cataract surgery).

1. *Absorbable sutures* eventually disappear from the tissues by foreign body reaction and digestion by macrophage cells. The commonest material has been catgut, which is prepared from the collagen of sheep's intestines by a comprehensive process of washing, cleaning and sterilisation. Each batch is tested for sterility, tensile strength and pliability and must conform to international standards. Plain catgut is absorbed within about 10 days whereas chromic catgut, which has been treated by chromic salts, takes up to 20 days to be absorbed. In eye surgery the tissues are not often under significant tension and plain catgut is mainly used in a grade of between 3/0 to 6/0 (2·5 to 1·0 metric). Recently plain collagen has been marketed; this is collagen prepared from tendons and is smoother and stronger (for equal calibre) than catgut. Polyglycolic acid (Dexon) is an absorbable synthetic polymer available in grades 4/0 to 7/0 (1·5 to 0·5 metric) and produces a minimal tissue reaction.

2. *Non-absorbable sutures* remain permanently in the tissues unless removed and usually produce little or no tissue reaction. Silk is

produced from the cocoon of the silkworm larvae. It is cleaned, processed, serum-proofed and sterilised and forms a strong and pliable thread. It is usually braided, but for intra-ocular surgery a fine virgin silk thread (8/0 or 0·4 metric) is frequently used as it combines sufficient strength with a fine calibre. Linen and cotton are not used much in eye surgery now as the synthetic polymers offer a more consistent strength and flexibility with the fine calibre required. Mersilene is made from terylyne; it is inert, strong, and serum-proofed. Polyester fibre (Dacron, Orlon, Ethiflex) is commonly used in eye surgery as it forms fibre which is strong, fine, non-capillary, and inert for the tissues.

ELECTRICAL EQUIPMENT AND ITS CARE

The modern operating theatre contains many types of electrical equipment:

1. Lights may be operated at mains *voltage* (240 volts) as most ceiling lights are; at 24 to 6 volts through a transformer, as many spot-lights and 'mains' ophthalmoscopes are; or by battery, as most hand-held lights and ophthalmoscopes are.

2. Electric motors are mains connected and are used to drive pumps and create pressure or suction as for example ventilation fans and suction cannula.

3. Electric solenoids and magnetic devices are mains connected and are used to control gas-flow valves as in the carbon-dioxide cryo unit. The giant magnet used to remove magnetic intraocular foreign-bodies is a large solenoid with a soft-iron core; the electric current needs to be rectified from alternating (a.c.) to direct current (d.c.) to prevent the rapid alternation of magnetic polarity which would occur at 50 Hertz (cycles per second).

4. Electromagnetic energy is used at a high frequency in the diathermy unit, which is also mains connected.

5. Diagnostic amplifiers with electronic circuits are used for producing the recording or visible trace of the electrocardiograph (e.c.g.) and the electroretinograph (e.r.g.).

6. Electric heating is generally produced through the resistance of a hot filament as with surgical cautery or in the heating of sterilising ovens and electric autoclaves. Since the cautery filament is in contact with the patient's tissues, it is essential that a low-voltage is used (preferably battery) as otherwise the patient would suffer a shock.

All electric equipment can be potentially dangerous, especially if it is connected to the mains; it is emphasised that for a mains supply with a stated voltage of 240 volts the voltage at the peak of the wave will be 400 volts and it is the peak voltage which can kill. All equipment should be under daily surveillance by the electrician, but there are several points in the care of apparatus which the nurse should know.

1. All mains-supplied apparatus should be earthed through the large pin of a three-pin plug. If the metal content of the apparatus were to become live, the electricity would pass to earth and blow the fuse. Fuses are easily melted segments of wire and form a weak link in the circuit; this protects the circuit and the person against damage from an electrical fault and no fuse should ever be replaced by ordinary wire or a fuse with a higher rating.

2. Flexible wires and connections become worn and are a weak point in the circuit, especially where they enter the apparatus. Any sign of wear should be reported for service, as neglected connections can become dangerous, especially if the insulation wears off and exposes bare wire.

3. The controlling knobs and switches on electrical equipment are subject to wear and can easily be broken. If this occurs or the control makes any unusual noise or buzzing sound, the equipment should be serviced.

Electricity is useful; it is also dangerous.

USE OF MAGNET

The giant magnet is an important item of equipment in the ophthalmic operating theatre, as it is often the only means of removing a foreign body from the eye, which could otherwise be blinded. It should be remembered that the magnetic flux is considerable and no watches should be worn in the theatre while the magnet is in use. Surgical instruments are also very easily magnetised and as far as possible non-magnetisable instruments are used; others should be removed from the field of surgery during the time the magnet is active. It is advantageous to prepare two operation sets, with separate types of instruments, the non-magnetisable instruments being laid on the same trolley as the magnetic probes.

There are two types of giant magnet (Fig. 8.14). The Mellinger is a solenoid which surrounds the patient's head and creates a magnetic field within its centre; the hand-held probe and the foreign body are both magnetised, are mutually attracted, and by careful manipulation of the probe the foreign body is directed and removed from the eye through the operation wound. The Phelp's magnet has a soft-iron core permanently incorporated in the solenoid, which can therefore be of a more compact construction; there are no hand-held probes, although

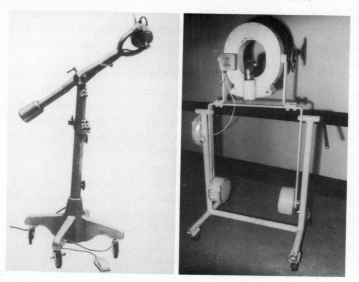

Fig. 8.14 Giant magnets – Phelps, Mellinger

probes of various shapes can be screwed into the permanent core and the whole apparatus is manipulated in order to attract the foreign body from the eye. Both magnets are heavy and need to be counterbalanced, but the Phelp's needs to combine this with greater mobility, and the joints should be carefully maintained and lubricated. Experience with the magnet is vital for the successful removal of a foreign body. All foreign bodies should be carefully filed and stored, as, in common with other injuries, many will lead to legal claims for compensation.

9

Care and sterilisation of instruments

ORGANISATION

The complex organisation of many sterilisation services arises from the increasing costs and the need to maximise the use of expensive equipment now in use. The *Listerean* revolution, with its emphasis on antiseptic and aseptic surgery, is one of the foundations of modern safe surgery and much research has been carried out to improve the technology of sterilisation. Many pathogenic microbes are not killed by antiseptic chemicals, and such chemicals are also toxic to the exposed tissues of the patients, so that almost all routine sterilisation depends on the application of heat over a period of time sufficient to kill all microbes. The heat must not be so hot as to destroy the instruments or other materials, but simple boiling in water does *not* kill the most resistant microbes such as tetanus and gas-gangrene spores. Sterilisation under the steam pressure of an autoclave or in a hot air oven is regarded as efficient but may damage suture materials or other susceptible materials.

The development of central (CSSD) and theatre (TSSD) sterile supply departments has occurred over the last twenty years to meet the needs of a higher standard of sterilisation and the increasing demands for supplies of surgical equipment.

Centralisation has several advantages including:

1. Maximising the use of expensive equipment.
2. Reducing the need for expensive and bulky equipment in every ward and department. Topping-up systems may be used and the daily requirements of each department monitored.
3. Concentrating the area of operation so that microbiological surveillance of sterile procedures can also be concentrated.
4. Allowing the training of staff skilled in sterile procedures to be specialised.

There are disadvantages, which may sometimes outweigh the advantages:

1. Increased costs arising from (a) transport costs, or (b) storage space required for packs, especially if CSSD is operated on a five-day week.
2. Reduplication of equipment in peripheral departments, when sterilised supplies are required immediately or where the CSSD is not operational.
3. Ophthalmic dressings and instruments are often small or fragile and can be damaged by the mass-processing methods adopted in a modern CSSD.
   Expensive instruments can be thrown out with the disposable materials, which predominate.

These and other considerations will occur to the nurse who has to decide if or how much to rely on a central sterilising department; transport and storage may incur liabilities as will the discipline of inventoring the sending and return of instruments.

STORAGE

The storage of instruments and packs will be within easy reach of staff in the treatment rooms and theatre. Instruments requiring sterilisation before use will naturally be stored within the same area as the steriliser, while sterile packs and other equipment may be stored nearer the patients' treatment chair or couch:

1. The instrument cupboard (Fig. 9.1) with glass-paned doors and glass shelves has been used over many years for the storage of non-sterile instruments. It has the advantage that the very large number of small instruments used in ophthalmic surgery can be stored in a fairly small space and within view when needed.
2. Transparent plastic boxes (Fig. 9.2) have replaced the black velveted boxes for the storage of individual instruments or sets. The instruments are more easily seen and their condition and identity checked. The boxes are useful for the storage of a reserve of instruments or for sending instruments through the post for service.
3. Open shelves are often used for the storage of the packs from the CSSD as these packs can vary in size from a sterile envelope a few centimetres square to a cardboard box with a dimension of several decimetres. Where a large number of packs are stored, shelves tend to be placed up to ceiling level, which makes access difficult and becomes a fire hazard; if a proper stock-control is not maintained, packs on the top shelf may be neglected and become time-expired.
4. Closed shelves (Fig. 9.3) are tidier and can be designed to

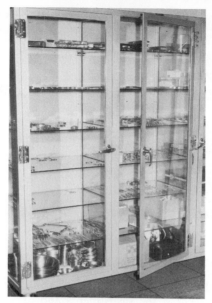

Fig. 9.1 Instrument cupboard

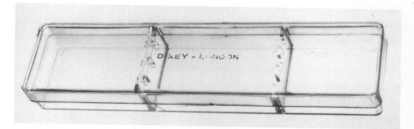

Fig. 9.2 Plastic container for instruments

accommodate standard packs, if the CSSD maintains a policy of standard sizes. Containers can be designed on the supermarket system in which the new supply is fed in at the end opposite to that of the user.

Storage areas require regular maintenance (cleaning, repair, painting, etc.) if they are to remain hygienic.

After use equipment to be resterilised can be discarded into a transport bucket of disinfectant solution for return to the CSSD but most ophthalmic equipment requires specialised cleaning and handling and is usually packed in the department before return. Disposable needles should be disposed of in special containers so as not to pierce the rubbish bag or cause injury to those handling it.

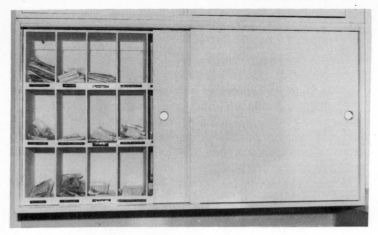

Fig. 9.3 Closed shelves

CLEANING AND SHARPENING

Sterilisation is the removal and destruction of all living microbes and can only be efficient if the instruments and dressings are cleaned thoroughly before the sterilising process. Residues of dried serum or blood will be coagulated by the heat and interfere with the use of instruments, especially at moveable joints. There are several methods of cleaning:

1. *Simple wipe.* Flat surfaces of instruments are best wiped clean with a detergent solution immediately after surgery and before residues have coagulated.

2. *Ultrasound.* Crevices and joints in the instruments are often inaccessible even when the instrument is dissembled. The cleaned instruments should be exposed to ultrasound in a detergent bath; the ultrasound vibrations are concentrated within the crevices and particles of dirt shaken out.

3. *Eyzyme.* Serum and lens protein is resistant to cleaning by ordinary washing solution and may be removed from drapes and gowns by using washing powders with an enzyme action (protamines).

4. The surface of operating microscopes, giant magnets, and some probes requires special methods as these cannot be cleaned and sterilised in bulk. The equipment must be cleaned thoroughly with an antistatic detergent fluid; dry sterilised handling guards are provided to cover any control knobs and levers.

Sharpening of instruments has become less important with the increased availability of disposable needles and blades, which are

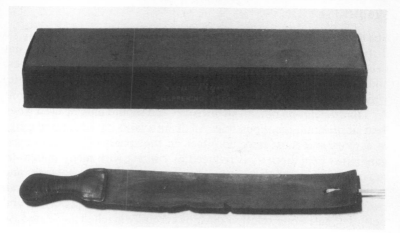

Fig. 9.4 Hone and leather for sharpening cataract knife

supplied in sterile packs and contribute to the ease of modern sterile procedures. The cataract knife especially requires to be maintained in a perfectly sharp condition and the theatre nurse may still find the moderate skill required in its maintenance useful. The technique is similar to that used for the old 'cut-throat' razor and requires a hone and leather (Fig. 9.4). The blade is sharpened along its whole length evenly by drawing it along the oiled hone on the flat of the blade's side and with the sharp edge trailing; at the end of each sweep the blade is turned over with its back to the hone and a return sweep sharpens the other side of the blade. After about four sweeps of each side the process is repeated on the leather, which gives a polished finish. Attention should be given to the point of the blade, which should be especially sharp but is also very vulnerable to damage.

Titanium alloys are being used in the manufacture of microsurgical instruments and aim to have some advantages over the usual chrome-nickel stainless steel. Titanium alloys tend to be lighter in weight, but harder so that the delicate teeth and sharp edges resist wear.

Microsurgical knives with a diamond cutting-edge are being manufactured for ophthalmic operations and are both extremely sharp and retain this sharpness after repeated sterilisation.

Other instruments can be sharpened such as keratomes and scissors. Trephines are difficult to sharpen to an even depth and are usually re-sharpened by the manufacturer. Disposable needles are of a soft steel and should never be resharpened; their re-use will also create a hazard of cross-infection for hepatitis virus.

STERILISATION

Sterilisation, which is the killing of ALL microbes, should be distinguished from disinfection, in which harmful microbes but not necessarily their spores, are removed. Surgical instruments, drapes, and dressing must be sterile and that equipment (such as plastic) which is damaged by heat poses a special problem for sterilisation:

A. *Disinfectants* do not kill all microbes and should only be used when heat sterilisation is not possible. All disinfectants have a limited range of activity and most have no effect on the spores of tetanus or gas gangrene. Their activity is reduced by contact with many materials; organic matter, swabs, some detergents, hard water, cork and polymers. Some organisms such as *Pseudomonas pyocyaneous* can continue to live in some antiseptic solution for very long periods and bottles of antiseptic solution must be carefully lavelled and dated, so that the storage period can be controlled; cork or stopper liners must not be used.

The *uses* of disinfectants in hospital can be irrational and many hospitals have now adopted antiseptic policies, which restrict their use. Such policies may:

1. define the indications for using disinfectants;
2. define the choice of disinfectant for each purpose;
3. limit the number of different disinfectants to the most useful and specify the dilutions to be used.

There are four main uses:

1. treatment of skin and mucous surfaces;
2. disinfection of instruments easily damaged by heat;
3. rendering relatively safe for handling contaminated and potentially infectious instruments and equipment;
4. decontamination of surfaces such as dressing-trolleys.

B. *Heat sterilisation* is either by the autoclave or hot-air oven, as the old water boiler does not reach a sufficiently high temperature. The manufacturer takes great care to design and produce efficient and durable equipment and the nurse is advised to take some time in studying the instructions supplied with it. Apart from the sterilising chamber, the equipment will include important monitoring indicators or dials which deserve special attention:

1. *Pressure dial.* The pressure is measured in the chamber of the autoclave as it is the pressure which, by increasing the boiling point of water, allows the temperature to rise to an efficient level (about 130°C). A failure of the pressure will lead to a fall in temperature.

2. *Temperature dial.* The holding temperature, at which sterilisation is efficient, should be marked and the nurse should

ensure that this temperature is always reached. Even so, the temperature of the chamber is not necessarily the temperature reached inside a pack, which should be monitored by the insertion of a Browne steriliser control tube in its centre; where the tube has not turned bright green, the pack cannot be regarded as sterile.

3. *Time Clock*. The hold time for sterilisation is dependent on the temperature reached (Table 9.1). The holding time may be incorporated in an automatic operating cycle, in which case it can be checked by a watch while the temperature dial maintains the holding temperature.

Table 9.1   Sterilisation holding times.

Method	Temperature (°C)	Holding-time (minutes)
Autoclave	121	15
	126	10
	134	3
Oven	160	45
	170	18
	180	7.5
	190	1.5

There are available instruments (such as the Cambridge circular recorder, Fig. 9.5) which measure the parameters of temperature, pressure, and humidity simultaneously. The measurements are continuously recorded on a calibrated circular chart, which is rotated at a constant speed by an electronic clock.

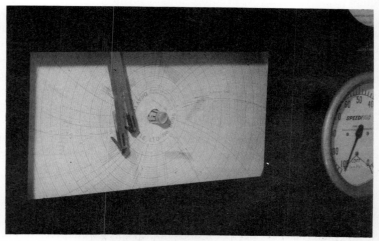

Fig. 9.5 Cambridge recorder for sterilisation

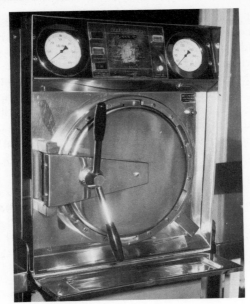

Fig. 9.6 Small electric autoclave

The modern steriliser is a sophisticated piece of equipment which will usually include warning lights to indicate which part of the cycle is operational; it requires understanding if it is to give reliable service. Operating manuals must be understood and instructions carefully followed; any defects will require urgent repair.

From the above considerations it will be clear that the ophthalmic unit will require at least two ovens for dry-heat sterilisation and this will principally serve the theatre unit; there is a British Standard (3421), which should be consulted. Most sterilisation will be performed in autoclaves, which can vary from the small types (Fig. 9.6), suitable for treatment rooms and casualty, to the larger autoclaves designed for operating theatres, and there are several British Standards (3233, 3970) referring to these.

'The autoclave is an essential item of equipment and its installation should include sufficient duplication to provide continuity of facilities while individual equipment is shut down for servicing.

SUTURES AND HEAT-SENSITIVE MATERIALS

Suture materials have been described in the previous chapter; they are easily destroyed by heat and are now mostly sterilised by gamma-radiation and supplied in sterile containers by the manufacturers. Once the inner sealed packet is opened, the suture should be used or rejected, but if the outer packet only has been opened, the inner can be stored in antiseptic solution.

Plastic materials are used in the leads of kryo applicator, diathermy and cautery equipment and these are easily destroyed by heat. Methods for their sterilisation include:

1. Low-pressure autoclave using steam at 80°C and formaldehyde over a period of 2 hours.
2. Ethylene oxide sterilisation with control of concentration of gas, temperature, and humidity.

Both methods need careful microbiological control using suitable test microbial spores (*Bacillus stearothemophilus* and *Bacillus subtilis* respectively) as well as the routine use of chemical indicators, which change colour. There are no British Standards for cool sterilisation, and a consultant microbiologist should advise on the choice of equipment.

TESTING PROCEDURES

Testing procedures are designed to check the quality of the instruments and of the sterilisation methods. All instruments need checking before sterilisation and this is usually conveniently carried out after they have been used and cleaned:

1. Macroscopic inspection is carried out in a good light using the naked eye and should reveal any major defect, breakage, or bending of the instruments. Spring elements in forceps and needle-holders should be checked by flexion of the instrument through its full range.
2. Microscopic inspection can be carried out using the low power magnification of a hand-lens (about +15 dioptres); this should reveal minor damage, dirt-retaining abrasions to the instrument's surface, or surface contamination with dried blood or serum. Higher magnification (×16) can be obtained with a low-power compound microscope (such as the operation microscope) and is used to ensure the quality of the cutting edge of knives and trephines.
3. Sharpness is checked by the use of a kid-drum. The drum (Fig. 9.7) has a membrane of stretched kid-leather or equivalent material, which the cataract knife or trephine should cut smoothly and with minimal pressure.

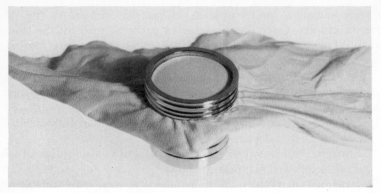

Fig. 9.7 Drum for testing sharp instruments

The testing procedure is completed with a check of the inventory of available instruments and the segregation of those to be sent for repair or to be replaced.

Sterilisation methods are tested by several methods, as indicated previously; physical, chemical, and biological indicators, as well as product sampling, have been used to monitor autoclave sterilisation processes. Physical indicators such as thermometers and pressure gauges attached to the steriliser, or melting point ampoules, will not monitor all parameters of a steam autoclave. All autoclaves should be equipped with time-temperature recorders to provide evidence of adequate sterilisation. A sterilising temperature maintained for an adequate time does not always achieve sterilisation, as a longer time will be needed if the load is dense or large volumes of fluid are present. Residual air or superheat may cause false readings. Chemical monitors such as test tape (scotch tape) or other heat-sensitive colour indicators are unsatisfactory, for they indicate only that the required temperature has been reached. Although product sampling may be the most reliable monitoring process for assuring sterility, it is impractical as a routine procedure for the hospital. Biological monitoring is accepted as the most effective method of checking a new sterilisation process or new apparatus:

1. Routine check of steriliser gauges showing the correct pressure, temperature, timing, etc. for every cycle of sterilisation.

2. Routine use of colour-changing tubes in every pack sterilised will check the penetration of heat into the materials, whereas colour changing adhesive tape only shows that the outside pack has been through the sterilising cycle. Browne tubes are in common use and are stored in the refrigerator to prevent premature colour change; during sterilisation they change from red to bright green according to the

temperature reached, and four types are distinguished by the spot colour:

I	Black spot for autoclave	change at up to 126°C
II	Yellow spot for high-temperature autoclave	change at over 126°C
III	Green spot for over	change at 160°C
IV	Blue spot for conveyor oven	change at over 180°C

3. Bacterial spore preparations can be provided by the microbiologist and are used in the development of new equipment or if the sterilising procedures appear to be suspect or defective. Spore-bearing strips should carry at least one million spores each and are essential in the surveillance of low-temperature formaldehyde or ethylene oxide steriliser. Steam and hot-air sterilisers should be checked once a week. Commercially available spore strips should be placed in the largest package within the largest load and never on an open shelf in the autoclave, or hot-air oven. Either the centre of the load or the bottom part near the exhaust valve, are the locations least likely to be exposed to sterilising temperatures for an adequate time.

4. Routine engineering inspection of equipment is required for the replacement of worn gaskets and for testing for air leaks. Sterilising equipment is subject to corrosion and wear and tear and requires a high standard of maintenance, details of which can be found in the texts listed in the Bibliography.

HOSPITAL AND CLINIC INFECTION

A natural balance occurs between man and the microbes, which are the small one-celled organisms responsible for infectious disease. Most microbes are not *pathogenic* and many are essential for the preservation of our environment; an example of these are the nitrogen-fixing bacteria associated with the roots of leguminous plants. Many of the skin organisms, such as *Staphylococcus albus*, are not pathogenic and others, such as *Staphylococcus aureus*, are relatively harmless until the skin has been penetrated by trauma or surgery or when the organism finds a nidus for multiplication such as the conjunctiva or a hair follicle. The normal protective barrier of the skin can be harmed by too much abrasive washing and strong detergents and the unwise use of antiseptics will kill the normal resident microbes and may cause more harmful microbes to replace them. Disease may also occur when the immune response of the body as a whole is inadequate; this occurs frequently with herpes simplex (cold sores and dendritic keratitis) and herpes zoster (shingles), when the virus may have been present in the tissues for many years in a latent (inactive) state. The immunity depends largely on a *clone* of lymphocytes producing adequate antibodies to control the microbe or virus.

The environment of the hospital and clinic is particularly prone to produce infection where patients with active infection are nursed, in the surgical wards, and in the laboratories where pathogenic organisms are investigated:

1. Self-infection occurs when the patient is infected by a microbe on his own body, as for example from the skin into an open wound.
2. Cross-infection occurs when infection is passed from patient to patient or from staff to patient. This may be direct, or during the dressing of a wound by infectious nursing staff, but is more often indirect through vectors such as air-borne dust and spray, medicaments, solutions and food.

Hospital infection may be particularly dangerous in young children, whose immune response is immature, and in the very old patient who is debilitated and poorly nourished.

The control of hospital infection will usually be the responsibility of a Control of Infection Committee, but much of the policy of control will be carried out by or under the direction of the nursing staff responsible for each clinical department. The precautionary measures adopted will depend on the degree of risk such as:

1. The operating zone within the theatre, where all materials and drapes will be sterilised up to the standard described in this chapter.

2. Barrier nursing for patients with dangerous pathogenic infection such as *Pseudomonas pyocyaneus*; this will include the separate disposal of used and contaminated materials. The separate laundering of bed linen will include a disinfecting period such as immersion for 10 minutes at 65°C or 3 minutes at 71°C, so that all material used should be purchased with the necessary resistance to this treatment.

3. Surgical nursing, such as dressings and instillation of eyedrops, should be carried out in separate treatment rooms where all work-surfaces are hygienically clean and the air fairly dust-free. On the ward all bed-making and cleaning should be completed at least one hour before any surgical dressing is performed, to allow for the settlement of dust and microbes.

It is difficult to maintain high standards of hygiene and cleanliness if the clinic becomes over-crowded with patients or cluttered with equipment; poor plumbing with exposed pipes or cupboards with flat tops create dust-traps, which increase the work of cleaning.

In summary it must be emphasised that all the modern techniques and apparatus of sterilisation will only be effective when the staff are concerned for the highest standards of hygiene and conscious of the dangers of hospital infection. Nothing does more to undermine this than an overcrowded clinic with poorly maintained equipment and plumbing and the accumulation of dust and dirt on the floors and walls.

10

Drugs as used in ophthalmology

Effect of drugs on the eye
Effect of drugs on disease
Diagnostic and other drugs
Routes of application
Treatment routines

If surgery seeks to heal the patient through the mechanical interaction of the scalpel and sutures with the tissues, drugs heal at the more subtle level of chemical interaction with the cells and their metabolic processes. The history of the use of drugs is probably as ancient as that of surgery, and drugs were often extracted by solution or percolation from herbs growing in the locality; some of these drugs are still in use in ophthalmology, including atropine from deadly nightshade and eserine from the calabar bean of West Africa.

Many drugs have a similar effect on the eye whether healthy or not, the effect depending on the chemistry of the cells or the transmission of substances between cells. Other drugs, such as antibiotics, are used, which have a maximum effect on disease processes or microbes but have a minimal effect on the tissues.

EFFECT OF DRUGS ON THE EYE

There are many drugs which affect the eye through interaction with the tissues, and some of these are shown in Fig. 10.1; more details will be found in the Bibliography.

Autonomic drugs
It was explained in Chapter 2 that, whereas the extraocular muscles of the eye (recti and obliques) are controlled by nerve nuclei of the midbrain and cerebral cortex, the intraocular muscles of the pupil and accommodation are controlled by the sympathetic and parasympathetic (autonomic) nerves. Mydriatic drugs, by stimulating sympathetic activity, produce dilatation of the pupil and must also paralyse accommodation (cycloplegia); miotic drugs stimulate parasympathetic activity and produce constriction of the pupil. (Fig. 10.1.)

Mydriasis is used to assist the detailed examination of the ocular fundus by ophthalmoscopy, especially when detailed examination of the periphery of the retina is needed. It is also used for fundus

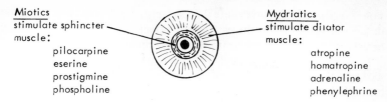

Miotics
stimulate sphincter
muscle:

    pilocarpine
    eserine
    prostigmine
    phospholine

Mydriatics
stimulate dilator
muscle:

    atropine
    homatropine
    adrenaline
    phenylephrine

Fig. 10.1 Action of drugs on pupil – miotics and mydriatics

photography and fluorescin angiography in order to maximise the light entering the eye and illuminating the fundus. In iritis mydriatics are used to prevent adhesions (posterior synechiae) between the iris and the crystalline lens; similarly a mydriatic may be used to prevent anterior synechiae to the cornea after a corneal perforating injury or corneal graft.

Cycloplegia is of most importance in the examination of the refraction of young children (under five years), who are unable to maintain fixation of a distant object and thereby relax their accommodation. It may also be required after intraocular surgery (especially glaucoma-filtration operations) to deepen the anterior chamber by increasing the tension on the zonular fibres of the lens.

Miosis is mostly used in the treatment of glaucoma. In most types of glaucoma and especially chronic simple glaucoma the use of a miotic eyedrop such as pilocarpine ½ per cent to 4 per cent results in a fall of intraocular pressure, and glaucoma can often be controlled by miotic therapy continued over many years or indefinitely. Miotics are also used to reverse the action of mydriatics, which may elevate the intraocular pressure.

Mydriatics

1. *Atropine* (0·5 per cent to 2 per cent) is a powerful mydriatic and cycloplegic drug, and is a natural alkaloid prepared from deadly nightshade (belladonna). After topical instillation its action may continue for up to two weeks and systemic absorption from the ocular tissues may result in a rapid pulse and flushed skin. Continued use of atropine may occasionally result in an allergic eczematous rash of the eyelids.

2. *Homatropine* (2 per cent to 5 per cent) is a derivative of atropine with a weaker and shorter action, wearing off within two days.

3. *Scopolamine* (0·25 per cent) is a powerful cycloplegic drug from henbane (hyoscyamus), but with a shorter activity than atropine, wearing off within three days. It is especially prone to systemic side effects and some patients become amnesic and disorientated.

4. *Cyclopentolate* (mydrilate 0·5 per cent, 1 per cent) is a synthetic mydriatic drug. It produces a rapid effect and wears off within 8 hours; it is therefore much used for examination in the clinic.

5. *Tropicamide* (mydriacyl 0·5 per cent, 1 per cent) is effective within 15 minutes and wears off in six hours. It is a good office cycloplegia for refraction.

6. *Eucatropine* (2 per cent to 10 per cent) is a milder derivative of atropine and has an activity of about three days. It may be used when the patient becomes allergic to topical atropine.

The following mydriatic drugs act like adrenalin by stimulating the dilator pupillae muscle rather than relaxing the sphincter. They are all mild and short-acting drugs with very little cycloplegic action:

7. *Phenylephrine* (2·5 per cent to 10 per cent) dilates within 15 minutes and wears off within a few hours. It is therefore in use in the clinic when examination of the fundus is required.

8. *Adrenaline*, neutral (epinephrine 0·5 per cent to 2 per cent) is a mild mydriatic. It also reduces the secretion of aqueous by the ciliary body and is used either alone or in combination with a miotic (e.g. pilocarpine) to reduce the intraocular pressure in glaucoma. Dilute solution (1 in 20 000) is used to whiten the eye in chronic conjunctivis, and may be combined with an astringent as in Guttae zinc sulphate 0·25 per cent c̄ adrenaline 1/20 000.

9. *Cocaine* is a powerful topical anaesthetic derived from the coca bush. It also acts as a mild mydriatic by blocking the re-uptake of adrenalin at the neuro-muscular junction. As its action depends on the normal release of adrenalin, it can be used to diagnose those diseases of the nerves to the pupil where the sympathetic release of adrenaline is defective. As an anaesthetic it can produce corneal clouding and systemic hyperexcitability, and it is therefore not much used.

Miotics

1. *Pilocarpine* (0·5 per cent to 6 per cent) is a moderately powerful miotic with a duration of activity of about six hours. It is used to reverse the actions of a mydriatic, after a clinic examination. It is also the miotic most often used to reduce the intraocular pressure in glaucoma, but after prolonged use it may produce a mild conjunctival allergy.

2. *Carbachol* (0·75 per cent to 3 per cent) has a slightly longer activity than pilocarpine but is less well absorbed.

Whereas pilocarpine and carbachol stimulate the sphincter of the pupil directly, the following cholinesterase inhibitors inactivate the enzyme that destroys acetylcholine; the effect of acetylcholine, which is normally present and similar to that of carbachol, is intensified.

3. *Eserine* (physostigmine 0·125 per cent to 0·5 per cent) is a fairly powerful miotic, but it often irritates the conjunctiva and is not used as much as in the past, before synthetic drugs such as echothiopate became available.

4. *Demecarium* (tosmolin, humorsol, 0·25 per cent) is a powerful miotic, but prolonged use tends to produce cysts of the iris which occlude the pupil. As with other powerful miotics, it may precipitate an acute attack in angle-closure glaucoma by obstructing the flow of aqueous through the pupil.

5. *Echothiopate* (phospholine iodide 0·03 per cent to 0·25 per cent) is one of the most frequently used of the powerful miotics. It has a long duration of activity so that it needs instillation only once or twice a day in comparison to four times for pilocarpine. It is used not only for glaucoma, but also to stimulate accommodation in those types of convergent squint which increase with the effort of voluntary accommodation. After being dissolved echothiopate deteriorates and should be kept in a cool place and renewed regularly within four weeks.

All powerful miotics should be used in the minimum effective concentration as they tend to induce ciliary spasm with myopia, retinal detachment and iris cysts. They also make the patient more sensitive to some relaxant drugs used for anaesthetic intubation, so that the anaesthetist should always be informed of their use.

Hypotensive drugs
In addition to the miotic drugs, there are other drugs which reduce intraocular pressure by either reducing the secretion of aqueous (e.g. acetazolomide) or by osmosis (e.g. urea).
1. *Carbonic anhydrase inhibitors* include:
   a. Acetazolamide (Diamox, 250 mg tablet)
                  (Diamox sustet, slow release, 500 mg)
   b. Ethoxyzolamide (Cardrase, 125 mg tablet)
   c. Dichlorphenamide (Daranide, 50 mg tablet)
   d. Methazolamide (Neptazane, 50 mg tablet)
These four drugs all inhibit the enzyme system of the ciliary epithelium and therefore reduce the formation of the aqueous. They are usually given by mouth, one tablet three or four times daily. After a week side effects may be noted, such as tingling of hands and feet, fatigue, nausea, and – rarely – skin rashes or kidney stones; many of these are avoided by the simultaneous administration of extra potassium in the form of potassium bicarbonate tablets or potassium chloride (Slow K, 600 mg).
2. *Glycerol* is a viscous liquid given by mouth in a dose of 1 to 1·5

millilitres per kilogram of body weight and is flavoured with orange or lemon. It is used to reduce the pressure in acute angle-closure glaucoma or before surgery.

3. *Urea* (ureaphil) is given by intravenous drip in a dose of 1 to 1·5 gram per kilogram of body weight to a maximum of 120 grams in 24 hours. It is effective in angle-closure glaucoma but any leakage into the tissues about the vein can produce phlebitis or even localised gangrene, so that the nurse requires to keep a close observation for this.

4. *Mannitol* (5 per cent to 20 per cent) is given by intravenous drip as a total dose of 2 gram per kilogram of body weight. As with glycerol and urea, it has a large molecule that draws fluid out from the eye by osmosis; these drugs have a diuretic effect and are contraindicated in liver and kidney disease.

5. *Timolol maleate* (timoptol 0·25 per cent) is a beta-adrenergic receptor-blocking agent used as an eyedrop and it has been used 12-hourly to reduce intraocular pressure without affecting pupil size or accommodation.

Anaesthetic drugs
Anaesthetic drugs reduce the sensitivity to pain, and most of the local anaesthetics used on or around the eye are synthetic chemicals similar to the natural alkaloid cocaine. These drugs inhibit the metabolic activity of the nerve fibres and block the transmission of nerve impulse; they may be used to block the transmission of motor nerves (akinesia) as well as pain or other sensory nerves (anaesthesia). Local anaesthetics may be applied topically as eyedrops to produce surface anaesthesia, or some are injected to provide a more widespread anaesthesia, as for the whole globe with paralysis of the eye and face muscles in cataract surgery. Cocaine itself is not much used now as it is easily destroyed by heat sterilisation and it also has many side effects including the production of over-excitability, restlessness, delirium, cardiac irregularity, and irregular respiration. Most topical anaesthetics and especially cocaine produce hazy opacification of the cornea after repeated instillation as eyedrops. The commonly used local anaesthetics include:

1. *Amethocaine hydrochloride* (0·25 per cent to 1 per cent) is used as eyedrops for surface anaesthetic.
2. *Oxybuprocaine* (benoxinate, 0·4 per cent) is also a surface anaesthetic but irritates less than amethocaine and is less likely to opacify the cornea.
3. *Proxymetacaine* (ophthaine, 0·5 per cent) is another surface anaesthetic used as eyedrops.

4. *Lignocaine hydrochloride* (xylocaine 1 per cent, 2 per cent, 4 per cent) is used as a regional anaesthetic by injection. As 4 per cent eyedrops it is used for surface anaesthesia.

5. *Procaine hydrochloride* (novocain, 2 per cent) is used as a regional anaesthetic by injection. As with lignocaine it may be combined with adrenaline 1 in 1000 to reduce systemic absorption and thereby prolong the regional anaesthesia. Procaine is sometimes combined with hyaluronidase, with assists spread through the tissues.

EFFECTS OF DRUGS ON DISEASE

The definition of disease as an aberration from a state of normal health has developed over the two thousand years of careful clinical observation and record since the Green physician, Hippocrates. Many drugs, mostly natural alkaloids, like colchicine in gout, were found to have a beneficial effect in reversing the manifestations of disease and had an established place in empirical therapeutics. The demand for effective treatment and cures has always exceeded the state of medical knowledge and there are many diseases for which no specific treatment is known. This is usually, as in iritis and uveitis, due to a lack of knowledge of the precise aetiological causes of disease and the history of medicine shows many speculative theories of aetiology from the humours of Greek medicine (blood, bile, phlegm and rheum) to the nineteenth-century theories of homeopathy, osteopathy and Christian science. In scientific medicine the nineteenth-century development of microbiology following the development of a germ-theory of disease by Pasteur and Koch has both rationalised the aetiology of infections and has led to specific chemotherapeutic drugs such as the sulphonamides and penicillin. In the mid-twentieth century the development of the *clone* theory and clinical immunology following the work of Burnet and Medawar has led to the use of drugs like the corticosteroids and azothioprine for modifying the immune response not only in infections but also in other inflammatory diseases and in transplant surgery. The role of histamine in allergy led to the development of antihistamines. The modern science of biochemistry has led to the use of minerals such as iron and vitamins in deficiency disease and to the use of hormonal treatment such as thyroxin in hypothyroidism and insulin in diabetes. Some of the disease controlling drugs used in ophthalmology will be considered.

Anti-infective drugs
Drugs used in infection are mostly chemotherapeutic and they may be

anti-bacterial, antiviral, or antimycotic:

1. *Antibacterial drugs:*

a. *Sulphonamides* have a limited range of activity, but are active against some important organisms such as *Streptococcus* and *Chlamydia* (trachoma agent), especially when given by mouth.

Sulphacetamide (10 per cent, 30 per cent) is used as eyedrops, and sulphadimidine (0·5 gram tablet) is used systemically. Sulphamethoxypyridazine is a long-acting sulphonamide used in a lower dose. Trimethoprim has been combined in a tablet (Bactrim, Septrin) with sulphamethoxazole; the combination is bactericidal and effective against a wide range of microbes.

b. *Antibiotics* have a selective capacity to inhibit bacterial growth (bacteriostatic) or to kill bacteria (bactericidal). Those commonly employed in ophthalmology include the penicillins (penicillin, methicillin, ampicillin, amoxicillin, carbenicillin), streptomycin, polymyxin, colistin, gentamicin and neomycin. Bacteriostatic antibiotics include tetracycline, chloramphenicol, erythromycin, and fusidic acid. (Fig. 10.2.)

All antibiotics have a restricted range of activity and the sensitivity of the microbe can change with the emergence of resistant strains of bacteria. Although it is often important to identify the organisms and their sensitivity by sending swabs in transport media to the laboratory, in many cases of infection immediate treatment is required and a selection of antibiotic is made on a basis of clinical probability. Many ophthalmic preparations include broad spectrum antibiotics such as tetracycline, neomycin, and framycetin, which will be active in most acute infections. Complications can arise from the indiscriminate dose, with the development of resistant organisms or a surface allergy to the drug. *Pseudomonas aeruginosa* infection is a destructive infection, which can occur after injury or surgery, and is usually unresponsive owing to its restricted range of sensitivity (to polymyxin, colistin, gentamicin, and carbenicillin); these antibiotics are not included in the commonly used eye preparations such as tetracycline, chloramphenicol and neomycin drops and ointment. The nurse will need to observe any lack of clinical response which may cause her to suspect:

(i) Use of the wrong antibiotic.

(ii) Inadequate dosage as when the patient has difficulty in applying the treatment.

(iii) Lack of penetration to the tissues as when topical drops are used for deeper infections.

(iv) Lack of immune response in malnutrition.

	Sulphonamide	Chloramphenicol	Neomycin	Tetracyclines	Erythromycin	Penicillins	Cephalosporins	Polymixins
Neisseria gonorrhoea	±				+	±	+	
Neisseria catarrhalis	+				+		+	
Haemophilus aegipticus		+		+	+		+	
Heamophilus influenzae		+		+	+		+	
Diplococcus of Morax–Axenfeld		+			+		+	
Diplococcus pneumoniae		+	+	+	+	+	+	
Streptococci	+	+	+	+	+	+	+	
Staphylococcus aureus		±	±	±	+	±	+	
Pseudomonas aeruginosa								+
Chlamydia trachomatosa	+			+	+			

+   effective

±   effective only sometimes

Fig. 10.2 Typical antibiotic activities

(v) Hypersensitive allergic reaction by the skin and conjunctiva.

2. *Antiviral drugs*

Topical idoxuridine (IDU 0·1 per cent) is effective against epithelial herpes simplex infection of the cornea (dendritic ulcer) if instilled frequently and early, before the infection has penetrated the deeper corneal stroma.

Cytarabine and adenine arabinoside have been given systemically for herpes simplex infection, but both are toxic drugs. Vidarabine (Vira-A) is available as a 3 per cent ointment for topical application to corneal herpes simplex, varicella-zoster and vaccinia.

The clinical cure of herpes simplex often depends on the patient's immune response, which may be stimulated by the intravenous injection of typhoid-paratyphoid vaccine (TAB 5 to 10 million killed organisms), which is followed by a short fever. Levamisole (50 mg) has been used in herpes simplex to stimulate the antibody-producing T-lymphocytes. Cauterisation is used in treating herpes simplex of the cornea. The anaesthetised cornea is dried and the infected area carefully painted with either strong carbolic (90 per cent) or iodine in an alcoholic solution; the infected cells with the contained virus are destroyed allowing normal cells to repair the ulcer.

3. *Anti-fungal drugs*

Polyene antibiotics include nystatin, which is administered topically, and amphotericin, which can be administered topically or be given by intravenous injection although it is toxic and side effects are common. Both drugs are active against yeast-like organisms such as *candida* (monilia). Fungal infection of the eye is rare but may occur as an opportunist infection when the immune system is depressed by disease or by corticosteroid therapy.

Anti-inflammatory drugs

Since the isolation of cortisone and its derivatives, such as hydrocortisone, prednisolone, and betamethasone, the corticosteroids have been used widely for their anti-inflammatory effects. Cortisone is a natural hormone of the adrenal cortex and many of its side effects are due to its normal hormonal properties, which are reduced in some of its derivatives. Prolonged use of corticosteroids, can result in water and salt retention, mental imbalance, hypertension, weakening of muscle and bone, delayed healing, hyperglycaemia, and, in children, delayed growth. The effects on the eye are more limited and include glaucoma, cataract, opportunist infection, and delayed healing.

1. Cortisone and hydrocortisone are insoluble and are not used so often in ophthalmic preparations now. The hydrocortisone suspension is sometimes used as a subconjunctival injection (10 mg) to produce a depot from which the hormone is absorbed into the anterior chamber over a period of one week for iridocyclitis.

2. Prednisolone (tablets of 5 mg) is frequently used by mouth when a systemic effect is required as in choroiditis. Soluble sodium prednisolone (Predsol 5 per cent) is used as an eyedrop either plain or in combination with 0·5 per cent neomycin (predsol-N).

3. Dexamethasone acetate (depomedrone 20 mg) is injected subconjunctivally to produce a depot as in hydrocortisone. As a 1 per cent solution (Maxidex) it is used as eyedrops or as a 0·5 per cent solution combined with framycetin 0·5 per cent and granicidin 0·005 per cent (sofradex), or as 1 per cent with neomycin and polymyxin (maxitrol).

4. Betamethasone sodium phosphate is used as a 0·1 per cent eyedrop or ointment (Betnasol) or combined with neomycin 0·05 per cent (Betnasol-N).

There are many other preparations with similar therapeutic properties, and used in a wide variety of non-infective eye diseases such as drug-induced blepharitis, phylctenular keratitis, pemphigus, vernal conjunctivitis, rosacea keratitis, insterstitial and sclerosing keratitis, many types of iritis, choroiditis or uveitis, sympathetic ophthalmia, temporal arteritis and retrobulbar neuritis (in multiple sclerosis).

5. Adrenocorticotrophic hormone (ACTH) is extracted from the pituitary and used as an intramuscular injection (40 units). It stimulates the adrenal to produce more cortisone and avoids some of the complications arising with systemic cortico-steroids.

6. Other non-corticoid anti-inflammatory drugs have been in use for a long time and include aspirin and its derivatives, soluble aspirin and benorylate; these are of particular value in uveitis complicating ankylosing spondylitis. Aspirin itself is a gastric irritant and may produce bleeding and anaemia. Phenylbutazone and oxyphen-butazone are anti-inflammatory when given by mouth. Oxyphen-butazone (tanderil) is available as an eye ointment for long-term use in anterior uveitis and scleritis and is free from the complications attending the use of corticosteroids.

Anti-allergic drugs

Corticosteroids are effective in suppressing the inflammatory aspects of many allergic conditions and have been the principal treatment of vernal conjunctivitis until recently. The conjunctivitis of hay fever and other sensitising allergies involves the action of histamine, which is blocked by the antihistamine drugs:

1. *Antihistamines* are usually given by mouth to control symptoms as they occur. They have been synthesised to a molecular structure sufficiently similar to that of histamine, so that they block its metabolic action in allergy, which is to produce dilatation of capillaries and exudation into the tissues as in the wheals of urticaria. Antihistamines are therefore most effective in the acute allergic conjunctivitis due to specific allergens such as pollen (hay-fever) or blepharoconjunctivitis medicamentosa due to topical drops such as atropine eyedrops. Antihistamines reduce the irritation and may be administered topically as well as orally:

a. Guttae otrivine-antistin is a topical solution used in allergic conjunctivitis; it combines a vasoconstrictor with the antihis-tamine.

b. Chlorpheniramine (haymine, piriton, 4 mg tablets) is given up to 12 mg daily.

c. Diphenhydramine (benadryl, 25 mg tablets) is given up to about 150 mg daily.

d. Mepyramine (anthisan, 50 mg tablets) is given up to 400 mg daily.

e. Phenindamine tartrate (thephorin 25 mg tablets) is given up to 600 mg daily and, unlike most antihistamines, does not produce drowsiness.

f. Promethazine (promethrax, phenergan 10 or 25 mg tablets) is given 25 mg at night and 10 mg by day.

g. Trimeprazine (vallergan, 10 mg) is given more for its sedative action than as an antihistamine.

The above drugs would be prescribed in a lower dose to children and most are available in an elixir preparation.

2. *Sodium cromoglycate* (opticrom eyedrops, 2 per cent) are instilled three to four times daily in allergic conjunctivitis, particularly vernal catarrh.

3. *Corticosteroid* eyedrops and ointment (such as prednisolone, betamethasone) are used in allergic conditions for their anti-allergic properties; although they will improve the symptoms, they may reduce the local immunity to infection.

4. *Desensitizing vaccines* are sometimes used to block the action of the allergy-producing antigen. If the history suggests a specific type of antigen, such as pollen in hayfever, this may be confirmed by the reaction produced by the skin on a scratch-test using pollen solutions. Multidose vials of vaccine may be ordered, prepared from pollen, house-mite, or other allergens, and the patient receives a course of injections at gradually increasing doses. Allergic reactions occasionally occur and the nurse should always include a vial of adrenaline injection 0·1 per cent B.P., with the set; minor reactions can be covered by an antihistamine.

DIAGNOSTIC DRUGS

Disease of the cornea may be demonstrated by the use of vital-stains, the commonest being:

1. Fluorescin eyedrops 2 per cent, which is instilled and washed away with saline. It is useful for demonstrating gaps in the corneal epithelium and corneal abrasions and is also used in applanation tonometry to stain the corneal fluid. Diluted with saline it shows up green and the fluorescent effect is intensified by the using of light from a cobalt-blue filter.

2. Rose Bengal eyedrops 1 per cent which are instilled without dilution, the excess being mopped away. Rose Bengal stains diseased cells as in herpes simplex keratitis, corneal ulceration, and keratoconjunctivitis sicca (dry-eye syndrome).

OTHER DRUGS IN OPHTHALMOLOGY

Apart from ophthalmic preparations, many drugs of general application are used:

1. Analgesic drugs such as aspirin, paracetamide, pethidine and morphine are prescribed to relieve pain after surgery or in painful conditions such as severe glaucoma and uveitis.

2. Hormones include thyroid which may be prescribed in some cases of exophthalmos associated with hyperthyroidism. Most cases of *exophthalmos* (Grave's disease) are associated with hyperthyroidism and in these cases antithyroid drugs are often prescribed; these often intensify the eye signs of the disease.

3. Chelating agents help to remove insoluble salts, and in corneal burns due to lime, sodium versonate solution (2·7 per cent) may be used as an irrigation to prevent the precipitation of insoluble calcium salt. In most chemical burns immediate irrigation with water or saline is more important and the chelating agents are usually only available in factories where lime is in frequent production or use.

ROUTES OF APPLICATION

Ophthalmic drugs are frequently applied topically to the eye by solution in eyedrops or in an ointment. The efficacy of such preparations depends on a wide contact with the tissues and an absorption into the tissues of the eye. It happens that many of the original drugs used in this way, such as atropine, are readily absorbed and effective. The cornea, although only about 0·5 mm thick, is a complex structure of stromal connective tissue sandwiched between epithelial layers, so that the chemical transport systems required for the absorption of drugs are necessarily complicated, and the mechanisms depend partly on the chemical nature of the drug (for instance its solubility, its dispersal, its acidity or its molecular size).

Many drugs, such as the original cortisones, are poorly soluble and not absorbed, and for these drugs a subconjunctival injection may be more effective. Subconjunctival injection is also used when a high dose is required in the anterior chamber fairly quickly as with the injection of framycetin for intra-ocular infection.

Injection into the eye itself is of limited value and can be dangerous. It is therefore a surgical procedure. Sterile air, saline, or fluid silicon are occasionally injected into the posterior segment of the eye to reposition the retina in operations for retinal detachment.

Systemic absorption is required for most drugs acting on the tissue of the posterior of the eye and in choroiditis, for instance, antibiotics and corticosteroids would be given by mouth or intramuscular injection. There is a barrier to the absorption of many drugs into the

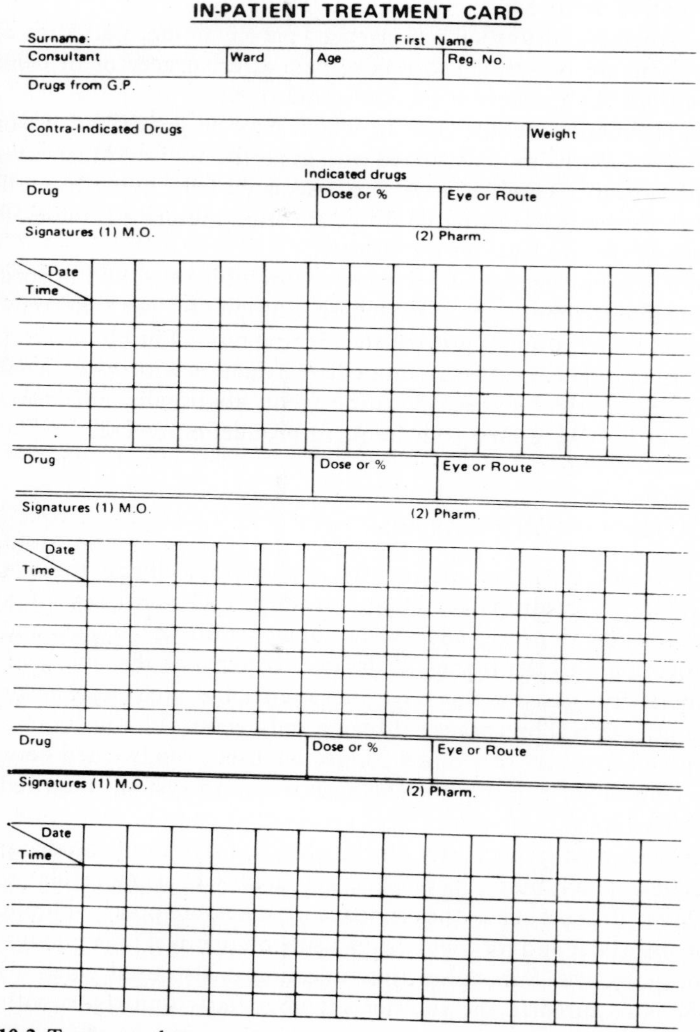

IN-PATIENT TREATMENT CARD

Surname:			First Name		
Consultant		Ward	Age		Reg. No.
Drugs from G.P.					

Contra-Indicated Drugs		Weight

Indicated drugs		
Drug	Dose or %	Eye or Route

Signatures (1) M.O.   (2) Pharm.

Date
Time

Drug | Dose or % | Eye or Route

Signatures (1) M.O.   (2) Pharm.

Date
Time

Drug | Dose or % | Eye or Route

Signatures (1) M.O.   (2) Pharm.

Date
Time

Fig. 10.3 Treatment sheet

eye (the blood-aqueous barrier) and this is the reason that some antibiotics are less effective in treating infections of the eye than elsewhere; sulphonamides and chloramphenicol are well absorbed, but the penicillins are not.

TREATMENT SCHEDULES AND ROUTINES

The problems associated with the effective delivery of treatment to the patient have been thoroughly analysed and go far beyond the simple prescription of the treatment and its dispensing. There are many factors in the non-compliance of the patient such as the mishandling of the drugs and the lack of insight into the need for regular medication; with ophthalmic preparations there is the added difficulty of self-administration, as anyone who has tried using eyedrops will appreciate. Most hospitals now use treatment sheets (Fig. 10.3), which record each administration of the drug, but these have not been accepted in domicilliary practice, where the nurse works more on her own and may be the only means of monitoring the effect of treatment. It is clear that the thorough documentation of all treatment is required; in ophthalmology a large majority of patients attend as outpatients and this documentation can usefully integrate the work of the hospital and community (domicilliary) nurses. The type of rules governing the control and storage of drugs has been given in the chapter on inpatient nursing and this can be adapted for outpatient and community clinics.

Hospital treatment can be centred on the ward's drug-trolley, which is moved from bed to bed and should have accommodation for each patient's treatment and the treatment sheets (Fig. 10.3). Most patients are mobilised early in theatre treatment or post-surgical care and much of the treatment is now centred on the treatment room. After each treatment the patient's treatment sheet will be marked for each *controlled drug* and the sheet will be signed by the administrator of the drug and a witness.

TREATMENT ROUTINES

1. *Instillation of eyedrops.* Eyedrops are a watery solution of the active drug in a vehicle, which may be water (single-use containers) or water with a mild antiseptic preservative (multidose containers). Once opened the drops can easily become contaminated and the date of preparation (with sterilisation) should always be checked.

a. Sit or lie the patient in a comfortable position with the head back but well supported.

b. Reassure the patient and explain each step in the routine as necessary.

c. Check the patient's treatment sheet against the label on the container and also the date of preparation and expiratory date, if included. Multidose containers can usually be used safely up to one month after first unsealing provided they are used on a single patient, sealed between use, and stored in a cool place.

d. Ask the patient to look up, place a forefinger on the patient's lower lid, which is gently drawn down to evert the lower fornix. Place the tip of the dropper about one centimetre above the conjunctiva and squeeze one drop into the fornix.

e. Ask the patient to close his eyes and use a gauze square to mop any excess that spills down the cheek. It is important not to exert pressure on the eye and not to damage the cornea by touching it with the dropper. Patients need to continue the administration of treatment at home and the self-administration of eyedrops requires to be taught and checked by the nurse. Eyedrops are produced in many types of container now (Fig. 10.4); the single-dose are useful in outpatients and surgical nursing, but multidose containers will be used by the patient at home. Slow releasing containers, which can be left in the fornix for up to a week, are a recent development.

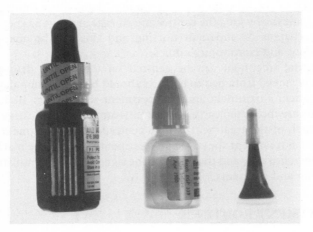

Fig. 10.4 Eyedrops containers – glass, plastic and single dose

2. *Instillation of ointment.* Ointments contain the active drug in either a water or oil emulsion. Ointments are not drained so readily by the naso-lacrimal duct, so that the medicament remains in contact with the eye longer. Ointments may also be used for their lubricating properties as in conjunctival burns, but their excessive use may make

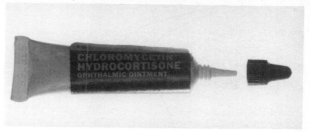

Fig. 10.5 Ointment container with application tip

it difficult to examine the eye or use an ophthalmoscope. The instillation is as for drops except that the ointment is squeezed out of the container (Fig. 10.5) along the lower fornix; the patient then closes his eyelids to prevent the ointment coming out and the excess ointment is wiped off the lids with a gauze square. Occasionally a glass rod is used to administer the ointment into the depths of the fornix; this rod should always be checked for any chip or roughness.

3. *Instillation of Collyrium and Irrigation.* Collyria are eye lotions and are less frequently used than in the past. Their use is mainly mechanical rather than the application of any particular drug contained in the solution, so that the only lotion usually needed is isotonic (0·9 per cent) sodium chloride. This is available in sterile containers and ampoules of various sizes for intravenous use and the same degree of sterile preparation is required for the eye; in an emergency, such as a chemical burn, a first aid irrigation may be performed with clean tap-water. A normal irrigation with saline lotion requires:

1 receiving dish (Manchester or Fisher's);
1 gallipot of sterile gauze swabs (about 10);
1 sterile undine (Fig. 10.6);
3 absorbent paper towels;
1 waterproof cape to protect patient;
1 lid retractor to evert eyelids.

a. The patient is sat well back with head supported or laid on a couch.

b. The patient is reassured and the routine explained as necessary.

c. The undine is filled from the sterile container. It has been traditional to warm the lotion to body temperature, but this is usually not necessary if the conjunctiva has been anaesthetised. The lotion can be warmed by placing the sterile container, still sealed, in a bowl of water warmed to 38°–40°C.

d. The eyelids are wiped clean of discharge.

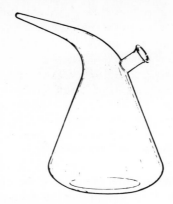

Fig. 10.6 Undine for irrigation of eye using collyria

e. The undine is poured on to the wrist of the nurse to check its temperature.

f. The dish is held by the patient or assistant against the cheek to catch the lotion as it flows from the eye.

g. The eyelid is held gently apart and the lotion poured in a steady stream on to the skin of the lateral canthus, then the lower fornix, and eventually around the whole conjunctival sac. The upper fornix is deep and it is usually necessary to evert the upper eyelid over the retractor so that the whole fornix can be irrigated. A gentle flow should be maintained throughout.

h. Finally the eyelids and face are dried with the swabs and absorbent towels. Any ointment or eyedrops prescribed will be instilled.

4. *Combination of treatments* are frequently required as prescribed for any particular eye disease. For example, iritis may be treated by a mydriatic, corticosteroid, and antibiotic as well as systemic therapy. In many instances the order of application is immaterial and it should be remembered that:

a. a second eyedrop tends to wash out any previous eyedrops if instilled immediately after.

b. Eye ointments should follow drops, which may be repelled by the oily base of the ointment.

Pharmacy

The principles of drug control have been referred to in Chapter 7 on inpatient nursing. The pharmacy is an important part of the hospital or clinic and will be responsible for the provision of drugs required by prescription and also those required for stock. Excessive stock is not required in the clinical department and any surplus or time-expired stock shall be returned to the pharmacy.

With commercial and industrial organisation more drugs are supplied in a factory format and it is only pharmacies in larger units with manufacturing facilities that will be able to prepare their own eyedrops in significant quantity. To avoid delays, the nurse should be observant of new trends in drug prescribing and inform the pharmacist who will be able to order stock to maintain supplies.

The pharmacist is a qualified professional, who should be able to assist the nurse in charge of a department if there is any query regarding the use or dose of any prescribed drug; it is important that he should be consulted as needed.

11

Ophthalmic nursing education

Ophthalmic nursing school
Development of ophthalmic nursing
syllabus
Ophthalmic nurse education and its
assessment

The importance of education for maintaining professional standards in nursing has been shown by the nineteenth century history of nursing outlined in the first chapter. The importance given to education can be judged by the larger number of nursing schools with full-time tutorial staff and by the concern to create a systematic theoretical basis to nursing (see Bibliography). Nursing is a practical art and its theories have been based on sound clinical experience tempered by the recent developments in social and management science. It continues to be a fundamental principle that all nursing theory should stand up to the facts of patient care and there must be a complete unity of teaching within both the clinical departments and the schools. Nursing theory divorced from practice soon becomes outdated, and theories are only validated as they stand up to the requirements and criticism of practical nursing. It is through a trained perception and disciplined emotion that the mature nurse will be able to achieve a professional quality of service to her patients.

THE NURSING SCHOOL

The facilities of an ophthalmic nursing school will vary with the number of students, but the range must be adequate and comprehensive. Ophthalmic nursing is essentially taught as a *post-registration* course and much of the essential basic sciences of anatomy and physiology should have been learned (in lesser detail) during the basic courses of general nursing. The school will therefore provide a training that shall be mainly clinical and the teaching controlled by those responsible for the standards of nursing care. The school shall be able to provide:

1. *Clinical experience* which is comprehensive and covers all the aspects of ophthalmic nursing described in this book.
2. *Teaching facilities* will include a building with lecture theatre and study rooms together with library. There should be office

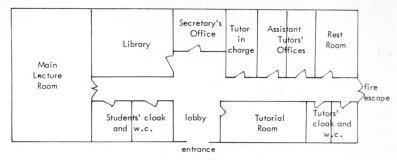

Fig. 11.1 Ophthalmic Nursing School – outline plan of principle facilities

accommodation for the tutors to organise the teaching and prepare their materials and lectures. Audio-visual aids may include cinematographic and slide projection, teaching machines, and closed-circuit television.

3. *Lecture and tutorial* timetables to cover all essential aspects of the syllabus as well as reinforcing knowledge gained by experience and clinical teaching in the wards and other clinical departments.

4. *Staff* will consist of classroom and clinical tutors experienced as well as qualifed in ophthalmic nursing. The practice of ophthalmic nursing is rapidly evolving and all teaching staff will need to keep abreast of the latest clinical methods.

5. *Recruitment* should normally be a responsibility of the school, which will need to extend knowledge of ophthalmic nursing to all those concerned in the nursing care of patients and to interest some sufficiently to join those courses of ophthalmic nurse education leading to a specialised qualification, such as the ophthalmic nursing diploma in Britain and Eire. Short courses in ophthalmic nursing for the general community and the industrial nurses promote a greater diffusion of knowledge about this speciality.

DEVELOPMENT OF OPHTHALMIC NURSING SYLLABUSES

The ophthalmic syllabuses are controlled in Britain and Eire by the Ophthalmic Nursing Board, which also inspects the schools and sets examinations for its ophthalmic diplomas and certificate. The syllabuses form a guide for the teachers and students, but cannot be as comprehensive as to include every detail of knowledge. As in science, knowledge is based on the data of experience and, as stated by Asher, clinical knowledge is based on observation, recording, and thinking. Chapter 3 has explained the need for accurate nursing records and thoughtful planning, but observation is biased and selective and it is the exposure of the student to work with those more expert and actively practising clinical nursing that will teach observational method. Nursing often seems to be treatment-orientated, but unless the nurse is taught to monitor the changes in the patient's condition brought about by treatment, nursing theory can become a method of justifying the treatments rather than an explanation of the observed facts. Just as a pianist must learn music by playing the piano rather than reading about it, so the nurse will learn most from her experience in the ward, clinic, and community, and the Ophthalmic Nursing Board has always placed much importance on the students' 'Record of Practical Instruction', which records not only that instruction in each procedure has been given, but also that the student has become competent. The contents of this record must be revised as methods change, whereas the syllabus gives a more general structure for the use of those implementing the training programme; this may be illustrated by part of the diploma syllabus, which is the training used for state registered nurses:

The Ophthalmic Nursing Board syllabus (1979)
The syllabus aims to provide the learner with a sound and co-ordinated knowledge of the theory and practice of ophthalmic nursing. A basic knowledge of ophthalmology is required, sufficient to allow the learner an intelligent understanding of the nursing procedures.

Structure and physiology
    The orbit – bones and surrounding structures
    The eyelids
    The lacrimal apparatus – tear formation and drainage
    The extraocular muscles
      etc.

Basic optics
    Light as a directed ray; reflection and refraction
    Role of mirrors, lenses, prisms
      etc.

Diseases, their investigations and treatment, involving:
    Lids and lacrimal apparatus
    Extraocular muscles
    Conjunctiva
      etc.

Practical nursing experience

This will be gained in adult and children's wards, accident and emergency and outpatient departments and theatre to meet the requirements set out in the Record of Practical Instruction.

N.B. Those undertaking the pre-registration course will spend a period of training on night duty.

Microbiology

Organisms found in and around the eye: pathogenic and commensal.

Taking of specimens for investigation; culture media.

Pharmacology

Drugs in common use in the treatment of ocular disease.

The effects and possible side-effects of these drugs.

Usual dosage and routes of administration.

Care and custody of drugs.

Special needs of ophthalmic patient

Mobility; escorting the blind patient.

Occupational therapy.

The role of the medical social worker.

Rehabilitation of the newly blind or partially-sighted patient.

Lecture requirements

The minimum number of lectures which should be given is as follows:

Structure and physiology	
Diseases of the eye	24*
Medical and surgical treatment	
Ophthalmic nursing – theory and practice	36
Surgical techniques – major and minor	
Pharmacology	4

* at least half of these lectures should be given by medical staff of consultant or registered specialist grade.

(The syllabus covers the different standards required for registered and enrolled general nurses and concludes with the examination regulations.)

This type of syllabus tends to emphasise the knowledge required and leaves the details of teaching to the expertise of the tutors. In practice the contents of the curriculum would show considerable overlap with those of ophthalmic assistant and technician curricula approved by the American Joint Commission on Allied Health

Personnel in Ophthalmology, and the differences reflect the much greater use of non-nursing assistants in the United States. It could be argued that much of the work performed by ophthalmic assistants is of a nursing nature and that the proliferation of new health professions is undesirable; on the other hand there is a need for nurses with an extended professional knowledge in many fields as well as ophthalmology, and when this need is not met by the schools of nursing the recruitment and training of technicians becomes inevitable. Curriculum development should therefore be a continuous process, extending the syllabuses to meet the needs of the patient. This can only occur in schools well integrated with the clinical departments and such schools should be able to advise on the revision of the national syllabuses.

OPHTHALMIC NURSE EDUCATION AND ITS ASSESSMENT

Modern learning theory has been based on psychological work performed at the beginning of this century before the discovery of the detailed facts of neurohistology and neurophysiology. It is obvious that learning must depend on the working of the central nervous system and its sensory receptors, particularly the senses of sight and hearing, but learning theory has usually adopted a 'black-box' attitude; in other words it analyses the organism's responses to a variety of stimuli without concerning itself with the intermediate connections (within the 'black-box' of the nervous system). A consideration of the retina as an information collecting system will by itself illustrate the complexity of this problem. Each human retina has about 135 million rods and cones responding to light and the resulting neurological pattern of stimulation converges on to one million ganglion cells, from which arise one million nerve fibres connecting the retina to the brain. The frequency code transmitting information in each nerve fibre can vary between zero and 100 impulses per second, so that the maximum information potential of two eyes could be 200 million bits per second (where a bit is the basic binary unit of information). This should be compared with a large electronic computer which has a central core capacity of about 250 thousand bits; in terms of information the retina of the human eye is a delicate mechanism with a capacity well beyond that of the most sophisticated computer yet built, and it is also much smaller and uses far less energy. Even so most of the visual information comes from the area of the macula, and the visual axis of the eye requires to be directed to the 'objects of attention', which could be the words on this printed page or those parts of the patient relevant to the nursing problem. The eyes and ears continue to search the environment for meaningful symbols; as in Karl Popper's 'searchlight' theory of the mind, the observing senses are directed to test the theories and hypotheses made by the observer, while in the 'bucket' theory, knowledge is accumulated as atoms of data absorbed through the senses. The commonsense theory is the basis of most theories of learning, in which knowledge establishes itself by the association or coincidence of data and ideas and the association is strengthened by repetition.

The psychological principles of learning were fundamentally influence by Pavlov's experiments on dogs and his concept of conditioned responses. Much of human learning is still described in terms of conditioning, but it should be remembered that Pavlov's experiments arose from his interest in the physiology of digestion and that human learning is not necessarily the same as that ascribed to other mammals in animal experiments:

1. Neurohistology shows that the newborn brain has an adult number of cells with very few of the adult *synaptic* connections, which develop during the first five years of life. This explains the comparative immaturity and dependence on its parents of the human baby, and the neurological plasticity, which contributes to the effect of early learning and experience on the adult pattern of brain-cell connections.

2. Symbolic meaning is especially important in human reasoning and learning and the same object, as for example a cross, may have entirely different emotional, religious, or material meanings according to the past experiences of the individual. The conditioning of animals is usually performed in artificial and isolating environments with simplified stimuli; these methods have been used in 'brain-washing' and are usually dehumanising as opposed to the humanising principles of some nineteenty century educationalists, such as Froebel. Nevertheless, classical conditioning experiments have led to a more careful definition of elements of learning such as re-inforcement, extinction, spontaneous recovery, generalisation and discrimination, as can be found in any elementary psychology text (see Bibliography).

3. The semantics of the verb 'to learn' have been distinguished by: 'to discover', 'to imitate', 'to make habitual' (Popper, see Bibliography). The last contains the minimum of discovery but clears the decks for further discovery, which may confirm or refute habitual knowledge if the nursing student has learned to critically assess clinical observation. Only the learner can learn and the teacher's role in this needs to be understood as a regulator, inspirer, or counsellor

rather than a repeater of knowledge and human textbook. The teacher should be able to check the student's understanding of the knowledge acquired and its conceptual structure. It is difficult to know how much teaching theory based on work with children can be related to adult learning, but it seems likely that Piaget's genetic epistemology should be understood, and especially his emphasis on the practical aspects of concept formation, which is closely linked to the symbolic meaning of language.

The student should find the study of ophthalmic nursing exciting not only as a means of widening her skills for the benefit of the patient, but also in bringing her into an area of knowledge fundamental to the learning process itself and to our concept of what is true (epistemology). It is obvious that for reading and ordinary observation, the eye is to man the primary sense organ and this is emphasised by the fact that the retina is part of the central nervous system.

During this century neurophysiologists, such as Granit, have examined the physiology of the retina and its connections to the brain in great detail and the tutor should be able to outline some of the effects of the physiological principles on the decoding of the images of external objects formed on the retina. The fact that all neurological information is transmitted in a binary form (nerve active or inactive, and synapse excitory or inhibitory) should be considered and the comparison of the eye to a television camera and monitor may be more useful than the traditional comparison to a photographic camera. The tutor may consider the following factors in an ophthalmic nursing education:

1. Syllabuses adopted will show that the curriculum can be divided into aspects best learned in the clinical situation and others learned in the classroom. The latter will mostly consist of factual knowledge from the 'laboratory' sciences (anatomy, physiology, optics, etc.) and it should be emphasised that simple classroom demonstration and experimentation is needed if this knowledge is to become more than a monotonous exercise in repetitive learning.

2. Communication between tutor and student should be two-way and can be facilitated in a tutorial rather than the traditional lecture system. Learning to communicate effectively by voice and pen is important to the nurse; it is also important for the tutor to adjust the teaching to the existing level of attainment of that pupil.

3. Classroom teaching will be used to reinforce the clinical teaching by emphasising principles of ophthalmic nursing (cognitive aspects), by elucidating any difficulties or ambiguity arising from the clinical teaching (error-elimination), by a control of emotional aspects of

ophthalmic nursing (empathic) and by inter-relating all aspects of ophthalmic knowledge within the nursing field (integration).

4. Clinical isolation is a danger of all specialised education and the tutor should emphasise the broader aspects of ophthalmic nursing and the way ophthalmic nursing embraces so many aspects of general nursing (e.g. paediatric, geriatric, diabetic, medical and surgical) within its practice. The student must learn not only to communicate to the patient and to the examiner – who will be expert in the student's field – but also to those nurses in the general field and administrators, who will expect to be instructed in problems outside their own background of education.

The *assessment* of ophthalmic nurses follows techniques common in education, and it is well to remember than in assessing the student one is also assessing the tutors and the school responsible for that student's education. Various methods of assessment have evolved including:

1. Multiple choice questionnaires (Fig. 11.2) which are all based on standardising the examinee's response to 'yes', 'no', or 'do not know'. The aim is to objectify the test, but it must be realised that even 'yes' and 'no' have different shades of meaning (as shown by an extraordinary variation of intonation), and that the method can only safely be used for testing factual knowledge without any ambiguity. Ophthalmology is a rapidly developing field and it may be difficult for the questionnaire to keep up to date.

TIME ALLOWED:–   1 hour

Select the most appropriate answer and tick in the right hand column.

1.   What important complication results from ocular contusion ?

     a.   Infection of the eye
     b.   Hyphaemia
     c.   Corneal scarring
     d.   Diplopia
     e.   All the above

2.   What is the main blood vessel supplying the eye called?

     a.   Ophthalmic vein
     b.   Central optic artery
     c.   Ciliary artery
     d.   Ophthalmic artery
     e.   Central ocular vein

3.   What is tested by the Ishihara Test

     a.   Colour vision
     b.   Reading vision
     c.   Field of vision
     d.   Childrens' vision
     e.   Stereopsis

4.   ....etc.

Fig. 11.2 Multiple choice question paper

2. Structured papers (Fig. 11.3) which allow for brief essay type answers but allow the examinee to spend most time on those parts of

the paper with the largest number of marks. It is a compromise between the multiple choice and the essay.

TIME ALLOWED 2 hours

IMPORTANT: Read the questions carefully and answer only what is asked as no marks will be given for irrelevant matter.
The maximum possible marks for each section of a question are indicated in the right hand margin.

MEDICAL SECTION

TWO QUESTIONS ONLY from this section to be answered.

1.	Describe how you would assess the visual acuity in the young and illiterate.	10 marks
	Discuss amblyopia in children and its treatment.	15 marks
2.	Write notes on:	
	a. virus conjunctivitis	10 marks
	b. virus keratitis	10 marks
	c. How do viruses differ from bacteria?	5 marks
3.	Describe the main features of retinal disease.	10 marks
	Elaborate the distinctive diagnostic appearances in three types of retinopathy and indicate briefly appropriate treatment.	15 marks

NURSING SECTION

TWO QUESTIONS ONLY from this section to be answered.

1.	Give the reasons for removing and eye.	6 marks
	What types of operations may be performed?	5 marks
	Describe the post-operative nursing care and the advice given to the patient on discharge from hospital.	14 marks
2.	Write short notes on the following:	
	a. Diamox	5 marks
	b. Idoxuridine (I.D.U., Keracid)	5 marks
	c. Trichiasis	5 marks
	d. Pterygium	5 marks
	e. Schirmer's Test	5 marks
ⅹ 3.	Early ambulation is practised in the post-operative care of ophthalmic patients.	
	a. Discuss the merits of this routine .	15 marks
	b. Give any contraindications .	10 marks

Fig. 11.3 Structured question paper

3. Essay papers (Fig. 11.4) which contain questions demanding not only factual knowledge but the ability to relate the facts within a logical framework and discuss their relevance. Each essay demands more than the other methods from the examinee and the marking can be subjective. It is important that the examiner is given guidelines as to the essential content expected, and the way the essay should be marked. It is the traditional method and may well endure, while the multiple choice questionnaire will continue to be used for more elementary assessments.

4. Oral assessment which is used to measure the examinee's abilities within the practice of nursing with a patient. The assessment will be based on the quality of the nursing routines used, and the ability to communicate with the patient and the examiner. This method is also subjective and precise guidelines need to be given to the

IMPORTANT: Read the questions carefully and answer only what is asked for, as no marks will be given for irrelevant matter.

TWO questions ONLY from each section must be answered.

TIME ALLOWED :- 2 hours

SECTION A
MEDICAL

1. How would you recognise that a patient, Mr. Smith, was developing sympathetic ophthalmitis, after corneal perforating injury?
   What is the treatment?
   How can it be prevented?

2. Write on FOUR of the following:-

   a. binocular vision
   b. spastic entropion
   c. presbyopia
   d. dendritic ulcer
   e. amblyopia ex anopsia

3. What is meant by a concomitant strabismus?
   What could be the cause?
   Describe the investigations and treatment which may be carried out on a four year old child, Victoria, who has a concomitant strabismus.

SECTION B
SURGICAL AND NURSING

1. Mrs Jones, aged 30 years, has been admitted to your ward, with a superior retinal detachment of her left eye.
   Describe:-

   a. the anatomy of the retina
   b. two causes of retinal detachment, and
   c. the pre-operative treatment and nursing care of Mrs. Jones.

2. Describe, in detail, TWO of the following procedures:-
   a. application of hot fomentation
   b. first dressing after a needling operation
   c. giving of a sub-conjuctival injection of Mydricaine.

3. How would you recognize that a patient may be a candidate for acute closed-angle glaucoma?
   What investigations may be done ?
   What treatment may be carried out?

Fig. 11.4 Essay question paper

examiner, who will also take into account the varying effect of examination stress on the examinee.

12

Ophthalmic nursing management

The professional nurse will know that management starts with the patient and his needs. In this context the many books on business management written in recent years have more to do with ward management than would seem at first reading (see Bibliography). Business may seem to be mainly about manufacturing and marketing, but more essentially it makes use of resources to produce results according to the most likely opportunities. Similarly, a doctor and nurse will use such resources as are available to the hospital and clinic for the benefit of the patient in terms of improving his prognosis. Prognosis is an important basis of management in any business, which can fail if the management spends too much on a traditional but outdated product or policy. Health costs money and any individual or community can only afford so much; equally without health there can be no wealth (the *Gorgas principle*) as the community supports more of its invalids and incapacitated members. The richer communities can bear the cost of retraining and rehabilitating mentally and physically handicapped persons, including the blind and partially-sighted, but in most poorer countries they either become an added burden to the family or beg on the street.

In ophthalmology the diagnosis and prognosis is established by the doctor who also prescribes the treatment, whereas the nursing sister or nurse in charge of the clinic or ward needs to deploy her staff and resources for the best needs of all the patients. Excessive care deployed on one individual will not only take care from others but may indeed make the patient more dependent and prolong his recovery. Eye diseases are almost never mortal and the prognosis can often be set in economic terms (quite apart from any pain and suffering):

1. Children with a squint leading to amblyopia will have a limited job choice later owing to monocular vision.
2. Adults with eye disease may lose time at work owing to prolonged

disability such as herpes simplex keratitis, or become economically blind from diabetes or hypertensive retinal disease.

3. Adults in modern industrial processes are often exposed to eye injuries such as corneal and intraocular foreign bodies and molten metal burns; prevention and effective treatment contribute to industrial efficiency.

4. Retired people becoming blind due to retinal degeneration or untreated cataract will become a greater responsibility and economic liability to their family and the social services.

Modern technology requires visual judgment and exacting eyesight so that any nation with a large population of visually disabled people (as in the Punjab with *trachoma*, or Norther Nigeria with *onchocerciasis*) will tend to be economically retarded, and it may be important to direct resources towards the prevention of these disabilities.

Cost control is as much the concern of a nursing executive as her counterpart in business, whether finance comes direct from patient charges or insurance or government funds. To spend more on staff, materials, or time than is necessary for the total patient care is likely to divert resources, which could be used in the treatment of others. Much ophthalmic equipment and treatment tends to be expensive and the nurse must be able to relate their comparative costs and to advise on the purchase of equipment, such as instruments, on the basis of price as well as quality and previous experience with alternative manufacturers.

Waste is a major cost factor in nursing, where standards of hygiene, sterility, and drug control are immediately of greater importance. Lister's methods of surgery have led from antisepsis and asepsis to a cult of sterilised packaged disposable instruments and dressings, so that the modern nurse can spend much of her daily routine throwing away used and unused materials; all this creates a psychology for waste as being necessary. Waste is often justified on a cost basis by the salesman, who rarely includes the costs of safe disposal for contaminated materials or the cost of accumulating non-degradable plastic materials in the waste tips of our cities. Lister's methods led to a revolution in surgery but the transfer of such methods of high sterility to a non-surgical area, as has been done with disposable eye-drop containers for outpatients, can be criticised; the use of the single drop container means that the container now costs much more than the medication and the costs of eye treatment have risen proportionately. The executive nurse requires to be knowledgable in the control of waste and to have the support of her colleagues in the administration.

In the face of rising costs and tighter budget control many health authorities will have appointed special multidisciplinary committees to monitor costs. But a committee must not be an excuse to replace action by discussion and it will be obvious that the expertise of a committee is no greater than that of its individual members; the power of the individual derives from the moral and disciplined application of individual knowledge.

OPHTHALMIC NURSING AND THE NHS

Britain has had a national health service directed from a government department since 1947. The capital resources (hospitals, clinics, and knowledge and expertise) were initially taken over from the existing local facilities, but gradual change has occurred as well as various abrupt attempt at reorganisation. The Beveridge concept that a health service would, through better health, lead to lower costs (Michael Cooper) has not been realised and there is no doubt that a policy of zero price at the point of service stimulated demand, a demand which soon had to be limited by the introduction of statutory charges for medical and dental treatment and for spectacles. The NHS remains a virtually free service for inpatients (except road accidents) and the increasing costs have been borne by the taxpayer. Cost cutting has been attempted by ministerial decree and by restructuring management rather than at the sources of cost demand (the patient and his treatment) and this creates the dilemma between cheaper but effective treatment or longer waiting periods for increasingly expensive treatment. For effective control of her department, the ophthalmic or other specialised nurse requires to know the elements of the new managerial system, which was imposed at the time of NHS reorganisation in 1974 (Fig. 12.1).

1. The centralised control by the Department of Health and Social Security (DHSS) is promulgated through a hierarchical tier of regional health authorities (RHA) to area health authorities (AHA), most of which are divided into districts; these have the same boundaries as local government authorities. Although it was intended that patients should be treated within their own districts, these boundaries often cut across the main transport systems and some patients would need to travel past the hospitals of one area to reach those of the area where they live. The structure may be seen as designed for future rather than existing facilities, but it has immediately allowed for a common budget for hospital, general practice, and community medicine and most nurses are now

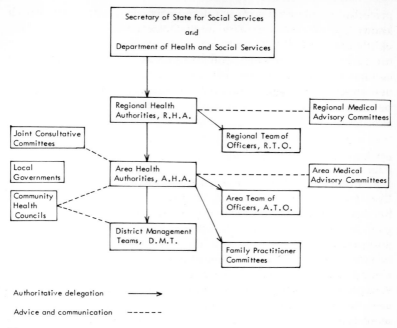

Fig. 12.1 Simplified structure of N.H.S. administration (England and Wales)

employed by an AHA. Similar arrangements have been set up in Scotland, Wales and Northern Ireland.

2. The district is administered by officers responsible to the AHA and a minority of these have direct clinical responsibilities. The management team includes a consultant, a general practitioner and the district nursing officer, administrator, community physician, and treasurer, and it is this team which is used by the authority to investigate and recommend changes in the use of resources, of staff, capital, revenue funds, etc. The team therefore has an ability to promote or restrict the work of those with clinical responsibility and all nurses with executive responsibility for wards and clinics will need to be aware of any actions taken by the team that may affect them, and to voice their opinion to the team as required. It will be seen that senior officers in the NHS now work more often as a team and there is less place for the senior officer making decisions as an individual; administration is on a basis of concensus after consultation.

3. Professional consultative committees are formed both at area and regional level so that the non-clincial officers and members of the authorities may be advised on matters they do not understand. It is only at regional level that there are specialist committees and the area

professional committees do not necessarily contain members with a knowledge of each speciality in medicine or in nursing, so that ophthalmic nurses will need to be particularly careful to keep the members of the nursing committees, as well as the nursing administrators, informed of all current problems in their departments. It is here that friction can occur between what seems to be clinically necessary and what seems to be administratively expedient. As the consultant ophthalmologist has the final clinical responsibility, the nurse may find that his interest in nursing problems can be of great value in any difference of opinion with the administrative managers.

4. Community health councils (CHC) have been a new feature since re-organisation. Although appointed bodies, the membership has been chosen to represent the patients' interests, whereas the membership of the area health authorities increasingly represents the interests of employees of the authority. Both the AHA and CHC members regularly visit the clinical units within their area and they will value and possibly use informed comment by the senior nurses; it is emphasised that they are not in a professional relationship with staff or patients and no clinical or privileged matters should be discussed with them.

This short summary of the structure of authority in the NHS can be supplemented by a reading of the 'Grey Book' and many nurses will have read the Salmon Report, which emphasises the separation of nurses with structural from those with sapiental authority and also created the basic models for the job descriptions now familiar to every senior nurse in the NHS. The future structure of the NHS may be modified by an increasing need for financial efficiency and it seems likely that in these changes those nurses with specialised knowledge and a wide experience will redress the balance toward sapiental authority. The British NHS certainly has problems as have all systems aiming at a comprehensive service of health care, but it does illustrate both the limitations and the successes of a service almost totally supported by taxation and with an attempted control by a centralised government department.

Within this service ophthalmic nursing is mainly allocated to the hospital eye units while most nursing of eye patients in the community is carried out by district nurses without ophthalmic training. When integration of services occurs, as has been the aim of the re-organisation, the ophthalmic nurse will play an increased role in both community and school nursing, which should lead to a higher standard; for the present it is essential that details of care are communicated fully when the patient leaves hospital so that the continuity of expert care and medication can be continued.

The ophthalmic nurse in charge of the eye hospital or eye unit should be a key person in the community and able to arrange courses of training for those nurses who need a knowledge of ophthalmic nursing (community, school, geriatric, industrial, etc.).

OPHTHALMIC NURSING OUTSIDE THE NHS

In Britain few ophthalmic nurses at present work in the private sector of health care as there was a tradition of all hospital patients being cared for in the voluntary hospital where they paid for treatment according to their means. The NHS has increasingly distinguished pay-beds from the others and the Health Service Act, 1977, will finally remove most ophthalmic pay-beds out of the NHS hospitals to private hospitals, where some ophthalmic nurses will find employement.

Industrial nursing at present contains the largest element of ophthalmic work outside the NHS and in most larger industrial cities eye injuries account for about 25 per cent of the total injuries sustained. It is important that the industrial nurse receives suitable training in ophthalmic nursing and maintains close communication with the NHS casualty department. She will use her knowledge to treat minor injuries of the superficial ocular tissues but know which more serious injuries to refer to hospital. Although responsible to the industrial medical officer, to whom she must report, her knowledge of ophthalmic nursing will be invaluable to him.

It will be realised that the patient will at times be treated within the NHS and at other times outside and the proper continuity of treatment requires good communication between professional staff in the various sectors of health care, whether by letter or, in urgent cases, by telephone. It can be extremely time-wasting for the receiving clinic to have to try to locate and communicate with the doctor or nurse referring the patient, and proper communication is not only polite but essential for the care of the patient.

In this book it is not possible to detail the methods used in other countries for the organisation of health care and the effect on ophthalmic nursing. Few countries outside the British Isles have specialist courses in ophthalmic nursing leading to nationally recognised diplomas, so that ophthalmic nursing is mostly carried out by general nurses who have acquired experience in this field or have taken a course organised by some of the larger eye hospitals. In these circumstances it is natural that ophthalmic nurses are not usually organised into their own professional group as in Britain, but international courses have been a means of bringing together nurses with a common interest in ophthalmology. A revival of interest in clinical nurse specialists is taking place in many countries and should lead to a better organisation of ophthalmic nursing as well as higher standards of care. As in Britain, the need for qualified ophthalmic nurses will depend to a great extent on the requirement of ophthalmologists, and this need may be reduced by the development of ophthalmic assistants, as has happened in the United States.

PROFESSIONAL RELATIONSHIPS

The relation between the nurse and the doctor in managing the care of the ophthalmic patient is mainly determined by the ethics of their professions. The nurse is professionally bound to carry out the treatment prescribed by the ophthalmologist and difficulties are unlikely to occur if this relationship is recognised. It is possible that a trainee ophthalmologist will often have less experience in the field than an experienced ophthalmic nurse, who should have no hesitation in querying treatment when she considers this to be incorrect. As long as this is done with proper tact and within an area of mutual respect, no difficulty should arise. Difficulties will arise if the nurse, because of her experience, begins to take on the duties and responsibilities of the doctor, which include the determination of the patient's diagnosis and prognosis. The adoption of a multidisciplinary concept of clinical management has sometimes led to a confused idea that the role of the doctor is not as leader but only as an equal member of a clinical team consisting of doctor, nurses, and paramedical professionals. The patient does not usually share this confusion, and attends the clinic or hospital with the intention of seeking advice and treatment from a doctor.

The doctor should respect the nurse for the skills that properly belong to nursing and will happily co-operate in allowing for the overlap of responsibility which occurs periodically. In the extended role of the nurse, who now performs many routine duties for the ophthalmologist such as urine testing, blood pressure estimation, visual acuity testing, and tonometry, it is important that she does not neglect her other professional duties, which are part of the core of nursing; in these the doctor will defer to her greater expertise and experience.

The ophthalmic nurse will also be in communication with other professionals, such as the orthoptist, refractionist, medical social worker, physiotherapist and occupational therapist; these are all expert in their own fields and will be treated with respect just as the nurse is respected by them. The ophthalmic nurse will also require to defer to her more senior colleagues, who will be more expert in administrative problems as she is in ophthalmic. While professionally equal, she may at times experience the problems of hierarchical control, which she will resolve with tact and by expressing only professional advice and opinion, deferring to her seniors in administrative matters.

Other persons working in the wards and clinics will include domestic, catering, and works and maintenance staff. These staff used to be responsible to the hospital and clinic administrators but NHS re-organisation has divided them into separate administrative hierarchies, each responsible to their own area officer. All these various staff will need to perform their duties within the constraints of the need for the patients for medical and nursing care and their work schedules require to be tactfully adjusted by arrangement between the nurse in charge and the appropriate supervisor of staff.

MANAGEMENT INFORMATION AND COMMUNICATION

In order to be informed, the recipient of a communication between individuals must clearly understand the language used. Communication may be considered in terms of the method or medium, the language, and the recipient person or audience.

Speech is the most frequently used method of communication, but it provides no record (unless taped) and can be unintentionally ambiguous; it is useful as a means of instant communication between staff or between the nurse and the patients, and may be used to reassure and to inform. The intonation of the voice together with any gesture has an emotive content and it is important that these relate accurately to the intention of the person speaking and to the words spoken; there can be nothing more likely to reduce confidence than a serious message given in an offhand and trivial manner.

Writing is the most important medium for permanent recording of data and messages and the clinical importance of nursing notes and nurse care planning has been explained previously (Chapter 3).

It is important to consider when communication between individuals should be oral or in writing; oral communication is sufficient for problems requiring instant solution, but the more likely that the problem is to extend over a period or require detailed considerations, the more important it is that the initial request is made in writing. During the writing of the letter, the nurse will be able to give time to a detailed formulation of the problems requiring solution and her copy of the letter will be a useful record of this.

The language of communication must always take account of the recipient and there is no substitute for a simple mode of expression as suggested by Gowers' *Plain English*. Necessarily within the profession a nurse will use technical jargon but she also becomes used to the simplification required when explaining to the patient details of the treatment required. She will also need to acquire a small vocabulary in building, plumbing, and electrical technology sufficient to explain her department's requirements, and a good dictionary will assist her in this.

The recipient of communication will not only expect to understand the language but will require the information to be relevant to his needs. The nurse throughout her training and experience will be particularly able to communicate at an appropriate level to the patient, or the doctor, but may find greater difficulty when explaining detailed requirements to the non-clinical workers in her department. There is no simple solution to this, but continued conversation will usually resolve any ambiguity; if the nurse knows something about the other person's work through experience or wider reading, this can be advantageous, and one important method is through the reading of the technical booklets supplied with items of medical and nursing equipment.

Nurses often find it difficult to explain a problem to a group of people with differing interests, as in a committee or a public address. In these circumstances the nurse should prepare simple notes, which she can use as necessary to speak on the problem and take sufficient data to answer any likely questions. The art of public speaking can only be acquired by practice and the nurse should not, through lack of experience, refuse an invitation to speak; always speak without haste and limit yourself to essential details without boring your audience with overlong digressions.

LEGAL RESPONSIBILITY

In a book on ophthalmic nursing it is sufficient to emphasise that the legal responsibility of a nurse arises out of her professional relationship to the patient as well as from her contract to any employing health authority, which may or may not bear the cost of malpractice insurance. In extending her knowledge beyond the requirement of basic nursing, the ophthalmic nurse extends her area of responsibility. The limits of this responsibility will be defined by the syllabuses of training for those diplomas which she has acquired and by the decision of the doctor to allow a nurse to perform any investigation or treatment. Insofar as these lie outside the syllabuses of training or are not special duties approved by the employing authority, the doctor prescribing the treatment may share a vicarious responsibility for the action of the nurse, and it could be that such duties would not be covered by the nurse's indemnity insurance.

Whereas a doctor's professional responsibility is limited by his willingness to undertake a patient's medical care, the nurse may feel that she is obliged to carry out the doctor's orders. Even though loyalty demands the acceptance of such orders, it may be a greater loyalty to the doctor to remind him of your lack of competence in certain procedures. The removal of a corneal foreign body, which used to be entirely the responsibility of a doctor, is now an established technique within the competence of a qualified ophthalmic nurse, but not other nurses who lack the necessary training. In Britain there is an increasing number of specialised nurses for disciplines such as ophthalmology and orthopaedics and this places an onus on the employing authority to ensure that their expertise is available to the patients. Staff leave and off duty schedules can only too easily combine to leave a junior nurse and junior doctor in charge of a situation and it is at these times that clinical disasters leading to malpractice claims have occurred. In a retrospective analysis the health authority may amend its policies, but written policies and procedures, however well thought out, cannot substitute for the lack of clinical experience and expertise of those professional persons directly responsible for patient care at every time of the day and night.

Bibliography

General
Bedford M A 1971 Colour atlas of ophthalmological diagnosis. Wolfe Publishers, London
Cashell G T, Durran I M 1974 Handbook of orthoptic principles. 3rd edn. Churchill Livingstone, Edinburgh
Martin Doyle 1977 Synopsis of ophthalmology. Wright, Bristol
May C H, Worth C 1968 Diseases of the eye. 13th edn. Ballière, London
Stein H A, Slatt B J 1976 The ophthalmic assistant. 3rd edn. Mosby, New York
Vaughan D, Asbury T 1977 General ophthalmology. Lange Medical, London
Wilson P 1976 Modern ophthalmic nursing. Arnold, London
Wybar K C 1974 Ophthalmology. 2nd edn. Ballière, London
Ophthalmic Nursing Board Prospectus. 1979

Chapter 1
Nightingale F 1970 Notes on nursing. Duckworth, London
Perkins E S, Hansell P 1972 An atlas of diseases of the eye. 2nd edn. Churchill Livingstone, Edinburgh
Woodward J 1974 To do the sick no harm. Routledge & Kegan Paul, London

Chapter 2
Davson H 1977 Physiology of the eye. 3rd edn. Churchill Livingstone, Edinburgh
Stephenson R W 1966 Anatomy, physiology and optics of the eye. Kimpton, London
Wolff E 1976 Anatomy of the eye and orbit. H K Lewis, London

Chapter 3
Inman I 1975 Towards a theory of nursing care. Royal College of Nursing, London
Little D E, Carnevali D L 1969 Nursing care planning. Lippincott, New York
Ross Woolley F, Warnick M W, Kane R L, Dyer E L 1974 Problem orientated nursing. Springer, Berlin
Stein H A, Slatt B J 1976 The ophthalmic assistant. Mosby, New York
Schappert-Kimmiger, Colenbrandes, Franken 1968 Coding system for disorders of the eye. Karger, Basel

Chapter 4
Chawla H B 1977 Simple eye diagnosis. 2nd edn. Churchill Livingstone, Edinburgh
Douglas A A 1976 Blindness from accident. Ross Foundation, Edinburgh
Gombos G M 1973 Handbook of ophthalmologic emergencies. Mosby, New York
Nuffield Provincial Hospitals Trust 1960 Casualty services and their setting. Oxford University Press, Oxford

Chapter 5
Becker B, Drew R C 1967 Current concepts in ophthalmology, vol 1. Mosby, New York

Becker B, Boode R M 1969 Current concepts in ophthalmology, vol 2. Mosby, New York

Blodi F C 1970 Current concepts in ophthalmology, vol 3. Mosby, New York

Nuffield Provincial Hospitals Trust 1968 Gateway and dividing line. Oxford University Press, Oxford

Nuffield Provincial Hospitals Trust 1965 Waiting in outpatients departments. Oxford University Press, Oxford

Ruben M 1975 Contact lens practice. Baillière Tindall, London

Chapter 7

Franklin B L 1974 Patient anxiety on admission to hospital. Royal College of Nursing, London

Perry E L 1974 Ward administration and teaching. Baillière Tindall, London

Chapter 8

Cranfield A B 1972 Theatre nurses handbook. Butterworths, London

Dorrell E D 1978 Surgery of the eye. Blackwells, Oxford

Stallard H B, Miller S 1973 Eye surgery. 3rd edn. Wright, Bristol

Various Instrument and Suture Catalogues including Davis & Geik, Ethicon, Dixey, Downs, Grieshaber, Keeler, Medical Workshop, Stortz and Weiss

Medical Defence Union and Royal College of Nursing, Safeguards against wrong operations. London

Chapter 9

Maurer, I M 1978 Hospital hygiene. 2nd edn. Arnold, London

Chapter 10

ABPI Data sheet compendium. Association of the British Pharmaceutical Industry, London

Ellis P P, Smith D L 1974 Handbook of ocular therapeutics. 4th edn. Kimpton, London

Chapter 11

Asher R 1972 Talking sense. Pitman, London

Bevis E O 1973 Curriculum building in nursing. Mosby, New York

De Cecco J P, Crawford W R 1974 The psychology of learning and instruction. Prentice-Hall, Englewood Cliffs

De Young L 1972 Foundations of nursing. Mosby, New York

Hilgard E R, Atkinson R C 1967 Introduction to psychology. Harcourt, Brace & World,

Mischel W 1976 Introduction to personality. Holt, Rinehart & Winston,

O'Connor K 1968 Learning, an introduction. MacMillan, London

Ophthalmic Nursing Board Syllabuses for diploma, advanced diploma and certificate. 1979 London

Popper K 1972 Objective knowledge, Oxford University Press, Oxford

Chapter 12

Cooper M H 1975 Rationing health care. Croom Helm, London

Fourcault M 1973 Birth of the clinic. Tavistock, London

Garrett R D 1973 Hospitals, a systems approach. Auerbach, Philadelphia

Luck, Luckman, Smith, Stringer 1971 Patients, hospitals and operational research, Tavistock, London

Lupton 1971 Management and social services. Penguin, Harmondsworth

O'Shaughnessy J 1966 Business organisation. Allen & Unwin, London

Pugh Hickson 1971 Writers on organisation. Penguin, Harmondsworth

Salmon Senior nurse staffing structure. 1966 HMSO, London

Schurr M 1975 Nurses and management. English Universities Press, London

Glossary

Abrasion	rubbing or scraping off; a wound (of skin or cornea) created in this way heals with the aid of medication; stitching is not necessary.
Accommodation	an adjustment in the focusing of the eye between far and near objects; uses the elastic moulding of the crystalline lens, which follows contraction of the ciliary muscle.
Adnexa	the accessory organs of the eye include the orbit, orbital contents, the eyelids, and the lacrimal apparatus.
Aerobic	organisms which require gaseous oxygen for life are aerobic; those that do not are anaerobic.
Albinism	a condition in which there is a lack of melanin pigment in the eyes, hair and skin
Amaurosis	a darkening of the vision; amaurosis fugax is an intermittent fleeting dimming of vision.
Amblyopia	a blurring of visual acuity without obvious signs of disease of the eye, as with the amblyopia of squint or toxic amblyopia (q.v.).
Anaemia	literally means the absence of blood, but refers to a deficiency of red blood cells and/or haemoglobin; it may produce a retinopathy (q.v.).
Aneurysm	a local saccular dilatation of a blood vessel, usually an artery; it may be congenital or follow disease or trauma.
Anterior chamber	the space between the back of the cornea and the front of the iris; filled with aqueous humour.
Aphakia	a condition in which the crystalline lens is absent, usually following cataract surgery.
Aqueous humour	clear fluid filling anterior chamber of eye.
Arteriosclerosis	a pathological thickening and rigidity of arteries found increasingly with age; it may result in retinal artery occlusion or in senile macular degeneration.
Arteritis	inflammation affecting the wall of an artery or many arteries (polyarteritis).
Asepsis	the absence of infection by micro-organisms.
Astigmatism	unequal refraction in different meridia of the eye; correctable by cylindrical rather than spherical lenses.
Atrophy	the wasting away of a structure, caused by malnourishment or lack of use.
Binary	characterised by or divisible into two parts or states, e.g. a neurone either transmits 'all or nothing'.
Bit	a unit of binary information, e.g. + or −, yes or no, and on or off.
Blepharitis	inflammation of the eyelid often due to infection but also to allergy or to the mite *Demodex*.
Blepharo-conjunctivitis	inflammation of the eyelid and conjunctiva, often due to infection or drug-allergy.

Blepharospasm	a tonic contraction of the orbicularis oculi muscle due to reflex irritation or to central stimulation.
Buphthalmos	infantile glaucoma (Greek for ox-eye).
Caruncle	a small, fleshy, pink mass; as seen at the inner canthus.
Cataract	an opacity of the crystalline lens of the eye; it will interfere with vision according to its size and density; commonly senile but may be congenital or acquired (trauma, diabetes, uveitis, etc.).
Cerebral aneurysm	an aneurysm (q.v.) affecting a cerebral artery, usually near base of brain; may produce cranial nerve palsy.
Chalazion	granulomatous swelling of meibomian (tarsal) gland of the eyelid.
Chelating agent	an organic complex which can hold metals (iron, cobalt, calcium, etc.) in a molecular ring by residual valencies.
Chemosis	oedema of conjunctiva.
Chlamydia	a genus of microbes taxonomically intermediate between viruses and bacteria; responsible for trachoma and psittocosis.
Chloroquine	antimalarial drug often used for rheumatoid arthritis; can cause retinal damage.
Choroiditis	inflammation of choroid caused by toxoplasma, tuberculosis, etc.
Cicatrization	pathological process leading to formation of a scar.
Ciliary body	that structure of the globe which forms the middle portion of the uveal tract; extends from the root of the iris to the choroid.
Circulatory shock	a depressed state of the blood circulation with low blood pressure and rapid feeble pulse.
Clone	a population of cells derived from a single cell by asexual reproduction.
Computerised tomography	x-ray showing soft tissue as well as bones by computerising an absorption matrix.
Concretion	a small white deposit in the conjunctiva associated with chronic infection.
Cones	nervous tissue which with rods forms outer layer of the retina.
Conjunctiva	the transparent mucous membrane which covers the front of the globe (except for the cornea) and back of the eyelids.
Conjunctivitis	inflammation of the conjunctiva; usually an infection but often due to allergic or irritative agents; such as smoke or occupational pollutants.
Controlled drugs	in the United Kingdom these drugs are subject to legal controls and available only on prescription.
Cornea	the transparent, circular disc at the front of the globe, through which the light passes and, together with the lens, is focused.
Corneal ulcer	necrosis of the anterior layers of the cornea, usually due to infection but also to exposure, corneal anaesthesia, etc.; stains with rose bengal drops.
Cryoprobe	a probe capable of being cooled to −70°C (200°K); used in ophthalmology as a method of holding the lens during cataract extraction and of producing a tissue reaction of the choroid in the treatment of retinal detachment; (also Kryoprobe).
Cryotherapy	the treatment of disease using a kryobrobe, for example small tumours of the eyelid.
CSSD	central sterile supplies department for the supply of packs of sterilised instruments and dressing.
Dacryocystitis	inflammation of wall of lacrimal sac; acute with pain and redness or chronic with mucopurulent discharge; treated by antibiotics or dacryocystorhinostomy.
Dacryocystorhinostomy	(DCR) an operation to drain the lacrimal sac by anastomising it to the middle meatus of the nose.

Diabetes mellitus	polyuria associated with glycosuria and hyperglycaemia; it may be complicated by a vascular retinopathy
Diagnosis	identification of disease by history and investigation.
Dialectic	a philosophical view of the growth of knowledge; thesis interacts with antithesis leading to a synthesis and new level of thesis.
Dioptre	a measure of the dioptric power of a lens calculated as the reciprocal of the focal length in metres (D = $^1/f$).
Diplopia	double vision; usually associated with squint, but may occur monocularly as with some cataracts.
Disease	disorder or illness of animals and plants (both physical and mental).
Ectopia lentis	dislocation or subluxation of crystalline lens; usually congenital or traumatic.
Ectropion	an out-turning of an eyelid due to a variety of condtions such as flaccidity, paralysis, and cicatrization.
Electrolysis	the separation of dissolved compounds into positive and negative ions by the passage of electricity.
Embolus	a foreign body (clot, fat, air, etc. carried in the blood and able to block the circulation.
Encephalitis	inflammation of the brain.
Energy	that quantity which has the capacity to work and defined as force multiplied by the distance.
Enophthalmos	recession of the eyeball towards the back of the orbit.
Entropion	an in-turning of the eyelid due to a variety of causes such as orbicularis spasm, trachoma, or injury.
Epilation	the removal of eyelashes, usually by epilation forceps; regrowth of the lash may be prevented by electrolysis.
Epiphora	an outpouring of tears, due to a fault in the lacrimal glands or lacrimal drainage channels.
Epithelioma	malignant skin tumour which may occur on the lid margin.
Exophthalmos	the abnormal protrusion of one or both eyes, mostly associated with thyroid disease; otherwise usually proptosis.
Exposure keratitis	an inflammation of the cornea occurring when the cornea is inadequately covered as with a facial nerve palsy, etc.
Extracapsular	in this type of cataract extraction the lenses capsule is opened and the lens removed from the capsule.
Fibre-optic	a method of transmitting light from source to instrument by a flexible cable composed of fine glass fibres.
Gamete	a sexual cell such as an ovum or spermatazoa, which unite to form the zygote.
Glaucoma	a disease characterised by an increased intraocular pressure and its consequences, mainly optic atrophy and scotomatous field loss.
Gonorrhoea	venereal infection which can produce conjunctivitis and iritis.
Gorgas principle	no wealth without health; William C. Gorgas (1854–1920), U.S. Army doctor, controlled yellow fever and made possible the Panama Canal.
Graves' disease	a disease characterised by exophthalmos and an increased excitability and tremor due to thyrotoxic goitre.
Hemianopia	a loss of half the visual field in each eye; homonymous if on same side, bitemporal if both temporal.
Heart failure	the output of the heart fails to meet the needs of the body.
Herpes simplex	cold sores, common on the lips, caused by a virus, herpesvirus hominus, causes dendritic corneal ulcer and diskiform keratitis.
Herpes zoster	shingles, a short painful eruption caused by infection of the sensory root ganglion by chicken-pox virus. It may affect the eye

	if the ophthalmic nerve is affected, producing a keratitis or uveitis.
High frequency	wave energy propagated at a high frequency of waves passing a point; low frequency audiowaves are less than 20 000 Hertz and can be heard.
Hodgkin's disease	a disease with chronic enlargement of lymph glands, spleen, and liver, and by anaemia.
Hypermetropia	longsight; a condition in which the image of an object viewed at infinity is formed behind the retina; corrected by a plus (convex) spectacle lens (q.v. page 34).
Hypertension	a group of diseases characterised by an abnormally increased blood pressure, and a retinopathy.
Hyphaema	the presence of blood in the anterior chamber of the eye, usually the lower part; often due to trauma.
Hypopyon	the presence of pus or an accumulation of white cells in the lower part of the anterior chamber.
Hypopyon ulcer	a corneal ulcer associated with an hypopyon; often due to pneumococci or staphylococci.
IDU	Idoxuridine BP, used in infection due to herpes simplex.
Interstitial keratitis	a keratitis with deep vascularisation of cornea; used to be common in congenital syphilis.
Intracapsular	in this type of cataract extraction the lens is removed within its intact capsule by rupturing the zonule.
Iridencleisis	a glaucoma operation in which part of the iris is brought out into the limbal incision to allow continued subconjunctival filtration.
Iridocyclitis	inflammation of the iris and ciliary body.
Iris	the coloured disc of the eye; visible through the transparent cornea.
Iritis	inflammation of the iris of the eye.
Intra-ocular pressure	pressure or tension of the eye; created by the secretion, flow and drainage of aqueous humour.
Keratitis	an inflammatory condition of the cornea, usually associated with a conjunctivitis; often due to bacterial or viral infection but occasionally to allergy, exposure (q.v. lagophthalmos), dry eye (q.v. kerato conjunctivitis sicca), etc.
Keratonconjunctivitis sicca	inflammation of the cornea and conjunctiva in a dry eye due to lacrimal dysfunction.
Kinetic energy	energy produced by motion of particles or any mass.
KP	keratic precipitates of white cells on the endothelium of the cornea in iridocyclitis.
Lacrimal gland	the gland which secretes tears.
Lacrimal sac	situated between eye and nose, through which the tears pass before entering the nose.
Lagophthalmos	exposure of the eye caused by incomplete closing of the eyelids.
Laser	a device producing light amplification by the stimulated emission of radiation; used in the coagulation of retinal lesions.
Lens	(i) the transparent, biconvex, avascular structure within the eye, situated behind the iris and in front of the vitreous. (ii) a glass or plastic structure, placed within a spectacle frame, to give clarity of vision.
Leucoma	a white scar of the cornea produced by healing; leucoma adherens has iris attached posteriorly.
Leukaemia	blood disease with a neoplastic increase in abnormal white cells.

Lime burns	corneal and conjunctival burns due to slaked lime; tend to chronic scarring and corneal opacity.
Listerean	Joseph Lister (1827–1912) promoted methods of antiseptic surgery based on a microbial theory of infection.
Macular degeneration	this condition, commonly due to arteriosclerosis, produces distortion of central vision.
Madarosis	absence of eyelashes.
Malnutrition	literally means bad nutrition, or undernourishment; a diet which is harmful to health.
Meibomian gland	one of a row of sebaceous glands opening along the lid margin.
Melanoma	a tumour containing darkly-pigmented (melanotic) cells; may occur in uvea, conjunctiva, or lids.
Migraine	a symptom complex consisting of periodic headaches often unilateral and often associated with nausea, vomiting, and visual flashes, etc.
Miotic	pertaining to miosis, i.e. constriction of the pupil of the eye.
Monocular	pertaining to one eye.
Multiple sclerosis	a disease caused by multiple, disseminated, and recurrent patches of sclerosis in the brain or spinal cord; often causes diplopia or retrobulbar neuritis (q.v.).
Mydriatic	pertaining to mydriasis, i.e. dilatation of the pupil of the eye.
Myasthenia gravis	a condition in which intermittent ptosis (q.v.) is associated with progressive muscular weakness; due to immune-block at neuromuscular junction.
Myopia	short sight, a condition in which the image of an object viewed at infinity is in front of the retina; corrected by a minus (concave) spectacle lens (q.v. page 34).
Myxoedema	the condition of the tissues caused by a deficiency of thyroid secretion.
Naevus	a birth mark, but often more specifically as a benign neoplasm containing pigment-producing cells.
Necrosis	death of a portion of an organ or tissue.
Neuritis	inflammation of a nerve (q.v. retrobulbar neuritis).
Nystagmus	a rhythmic jerky movement of the eyes from the normal point of fixation.
Onchocerciasis	a disease caused by infestation with the filarial worm, *Onchocerca volvulus*; often a uveitis.
Ophthalmia neonatorum	purulent conjunctivitis of the newborn.
Ophthalmoscope	an instrument for examining the interior of the eye by the observer looking along the line of the illuminating beam into the pupil.
Optic nerve	the second cranial nerve; it carries nervous impulses pertaining to sight.
Optic atrophy	atrophy of the optic nerve due to necrosis of some or all the ganglion nerve fibres and caused by conditions such as tabes, multiple sclerosis, tumours, trauma and points (methyl alcohol, tobacco, or quinine).
Orbit	the bony cavity within which the eye is contained.
Orbital cellulitis	inflammation of the cellular tissue of the orbit; often secondary to sinusitis.
Orthoptics	that science which is concerned with binocular function and the diagnosis and treatment of squint.
Panophthalmitis	inflammation affecting all parts of the eye; may complicate an infected wound.

Papillitis	inflammation of the optic nerve head, often due to multiple sclerosis.
Papilloedema	oedema of the optic nerve head, usually due to a cerebral tumour or cerebral oedema.
Paracentesis	surgical withdrawal of fluid from a cavity, as of withdrawal of aqueous from the anterior chamber.
Pathogenic	disease producing; often applied to microbes and other organisms.
Phaco-emulsification	surgical aspiration of a cataractous lens, which is emulsified by ultrasonic probe.
Photalgia	pain of the eye, caused by intensity of light.
Photocoagulation	coagulation by heat produced with a focal pencil of intense light; used mainly for dabetic retinopathy and for sealing retinal breaks.
Photophobia	abnormal sensitivity to light, usually producing blepharospasm; often due to corneal disease.
Pinguecula	a degeneration of subconjunctival tissue producing an elevated yellow spot near the limbus between the eyelids.
Post-registration	a term applied to nurses who have qualified and are registered with the General Nursing Council of Great Britain.
Primary care	health care organised at community level as opposed to hospital (secondary) care.
Proptosis	a forward displacement of the eyeball almost always a sign of orbital disease.
Pterygium	a wing-like triangle of vascular conjunctiva, which invades the nasal cornea, common in dry climates.
Ptosis	a drooping of the eyelid due to a weakness or paralysis of the levator palpabrae superioris muscle.
Retinopathy	a group of retinal diseases associated with impaired circulation, haemorrhages, exudates and oedemas, and often distorted vision.
Retrobulbar neuritis	inflammation of optic nerve.
Rodent ulcer	a slowly growing and locally malignant basal-celled epithelioma of the skin.
Rods	nervous tissue which, with cones, forms outer layer of the retina.
Rust ring	the infiltration around an iron corneal foreign body (q.v. page 83).
Sclera	the tough outer white coat of the eye.
Scotoma	blind area in visual field; arcuate scotoma arises from glaucoma.
Senile macular degeneration	a necrosis of the central retinal visual cells caused by arteriosclerosis of the related choroidal capillaries.
Serif	short line terminating each up and down stroke of a letter; non-serif test-type avoids these complicating features.
Sinusitis	inflammation of the paranasal sinuses; the pain may be confused with ocular pain.
Skialytic	a shadow-removing lamp using a wide distribution of focal illuminating sources.
Slit-lamp microscope	biomicroscope developed to examine the human eye and using a focal beam which can be reduced to a slit.
Speculum	instrument to expose the eye during surgery by retracting the eyelids.
Squint	condition in which both visual axes do not pass through the object of attention simultaneously (also called strabismus, q.v. page 97).

Stereoscopic vision	three-dimensional vision produced by binocular fusion of unequal retinal images.
Strabismus	see squint.
Stye	staphylococcal infection of a lash follicle.
Subconjunctival haemorrhage	bleeding between the conjunctiva and sclera; often due to injury.
Symblepharon	adhesion between the eyelid and globe of eye due to disease, trauma, and rarely congenital.
Sympathetic ophthalmia	severe inflammation in a healthy eye following perforating injury and inflammation of the other eye.
Synapse	one of the many junctions between the processes of interacting nerve cells; either excitatory or inhibitory.
Syphilis	a venereal disease with prolonged and varied manifestations; may cause optic neuritis or interstitial keratitis (q.v. page 107).
Temporal arteritis	cranial arteritis; inflammation of the arteries of the head in older patients with severe headaches and often terminating in blindness.
Tetanus	disease characterised by tonic spasm of jaw and other muscles leading to asphyxia; caused by toxin of *Clostridium tetani*, which enters by a wound.
Toxic amblyopia	blurring of vision due to toxins such as alcohol, tobacco, and various drugs.
Trabeculectomy	a glaucoma operation in which excision of part of the trabecular meshwork allows filtration of aqueous deep to a scleral flap.
Trachoma	chronic infection of conjunctiva and cornea by *Chlamydia trachomatosi*; gradual progress to scarring with entropion of lids and opacity of cornea, leading to blindness.
Uveitis	inflammation of uvea including iritis, cyclitis, choroiditis and panuveitis.
Visual acuity	the measure of acuteness of vision.
Vitreous humour	the gelatinous fluid which fills the interior of the eye posteriorly between the retina and lens.
Voltage	the electrical potential of a source of electrical supply expressed in volts where: voltage = current × load-resistance (Ohm's law).

Index